MANAGEMENT OF RENAL HYPERTENSION

Other titles in the *New Clinical Applications* Series:

Dermatology (Series Editor Dr J. L. Verbov)
   Dermatological Surgery
   Superficial Fungal Infections
   Talking Points in Dermatology – I
   Treatment in Dermatology
   Current Concepts in Contact Dermatitis
   Talking Points in Dermatology – II

Cardiology (Series Editor Dr D. Longmore)
   Cardiology Screening

Rheumatology (Series Editors Dr J. J. Calabro and Dr W. Carson Dick)
   Ankylosing Spondylitis
   Infections and Arthritis

Nephrology (Series Editor Dr G. R. D. Catto)
   Continuous Ambulatory Peritoneal Dialysis
   Management of Renal Hypertension
   Chronic Renal Failure
   Calculus Disease
   Pregnancy and Renal Disorders
   Multisystem Diseases
   Glomerulonephritis I
   Glomerulonephritis II

NEW
CLINICAL
APPLICATIONS
NEPHROLOGY

MANAGEMENT OF RENAL HYPERTENSION

Editor

G. R. D. CATTO
MD, FRCP, FRCP(G)

Reader in Medicine
University of Aberdeen
UK

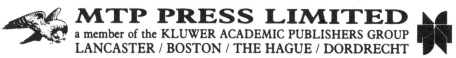

MTP PRESS LIMITED
a member of the KLUWER ACADEMIC PUBLISHERS GROUP
LANCASTER / BOSTON / THE HAGUE / DORDRECHT

Published in the UK and Europe by
MTP Press Limited
Falcon House
Lancaster, England

British Library Cataloguing in Publication Data

Management of renal hypertension.
  1. Man. Blood. Renal hypertension
  I. Catto, Graeme R.D. (Graeme Robertson
  Dawson), *1945–*
  616.6'1

Published in the USA by
MTP Press
A division of Kluwer Academic Publishers
101 Philip Drive
Norwell, MA 02061, USA

Library of Congress Cataloging in Publication Data

Management of renal hypertension.

  (New clinical applications. Nephrology)
  Includes bibliographies and index.
  1. Renal hypertension—Treatment.   I. Catto,
Graeme R.D.   II. Series.   [DNLM: 1. Hypertension,
Renal—therapy.   WG 340 M266]
RC918.R38M36   1987   616.1'32   88–545
ISBN 978-94-010-7067-6   ISBN 978-94-009-1277-9   (eBook)
DOI 10.1007/978-94-009-1277-9

Copyright © 1988 MTP Press Limited

Softcover reprint of the hardcover 1st edition 1988

Typeset and printed by Butler & Tanner Ltd,
Frome and London

CONTENTS

LIST OF AUTHORS

F. G. Adams
Dept of Diagnostic Radiology
Western Infirmary
Glasgow
G11 6NT
UK

V. E. Andreucci
Department of Nephrology
Second Faculty of Medicine
University of Naples
Via S. Pansini 5
80131 Naples
Italy

A. Dal Canton
Department of Nephrology
University of Reggio Calabria
  at Catanzaro
Via San Brunone di Coconia
58100 Catanzaro
Italy

C. Iles
MRC Blood Pressure Unit
Western Infirmary
Glasgow
G11 6NT
UK

P. J. Morris
Nuffield Department of
  Surgery
University of Oxford
John Radcliffe Hospital
Oxford
OX3 9DU
UK

J. A. Murie
Nuffield Department of
  Surgery
University of Oxford
John Radcliffe Hospital
Oxford
OX3 9DU
UK

D. Russo
Department of Nephrology
Second Faculty of Medicine
University of Naples
Via S. Pansini 5
80131 Naples
Italy

D. M. Tillman
MRC Blood Pressure Unit
Western Infirmary
Glasgow
G11 6NT
UK

J. Webster
Clinical Pharmacology Unit
Department of Medicine and
  Therapeutics
University of Aberdeen
Polwarth Building,
  Foresterhill
Aberdeen
AB9 2ZD
UK

R. Wilkinson
Department of Nephrology
University of Newcastle upon
  Tyne
Ward 4, Freeman Hospital
Newcastle upon Tyne
NE7 7DN
UK

SERIES EDITOR'S FOREWORD

During the last few years, renal hypertension has become a subject of increasing importance. The development of improved radiological techniques, notably intravenous and intra-arterial digital subtraction angiography, has made the diagnosis of renal artery stenosis more reliable, while advances in vascular surgery and the introduction of percutaneous transluminal angioplasty have caused major changes in clinical practice. The increasing use of such potent antihypertensive agents as the angiotensin I converting enzyme inhibitors has emphasized the problem of renal artery stenosis in older patients with widespread vascular disease as well as improving the prognosis of patients with accelerated hypertension.

This book examines the surgical and medical aspects of renal hypertension in the light of these recent advances. Each chapter has been written by a recognized expert in the field and provides information of relevance and practical importance to the average clinician. The developments of the last decade have emphasized that renal hypertension is no longer a matter only for the nephrologist but a subject on which all clinicians should be well informed.

G. R. D. CATTO

ABOUT THE EDITOR

Dr Graeme R. D. Catto is Reader in Medicine at the University of Aberdeen and Honorary Consultant Physician/Nephrologist to the Grampian Health Board. His current interest in transplant immunology was stimulated as a Harkness Fellow at Harvard Medical School and the Peter Bent Brigham Hospital, Boston, USA. He is a member of many medical societies including the Association of Physicians of Great Britain and Ireland, the Renal Association and the Transplantation Society. He has published widely on transplant and reproductive immunology, calcium metabolism and general nephrology.

1

MODERN DRUG THERAPY

J. WEBSTER

INTRODUCTION

Renal hypertension is not easy to define. Many forms of acute and chronic renal parenchymal and vascular disease may be associated with hypertension. Causation is more difficult to prove. 'Essential' hypertension may affect at least 20% of the adult population in Western societies and as a result will frequently coexist with other diseases. Furthermore, sustained hypertension, of whatever cause, results in impaired renal function. In the strictest sense, causation may only be proved if the renal disorder can be shown to precede the development of hypertension, and if the hypertension resolves after removal of the offending kidney or resolution of the renal disorder. This is seldom possible. Hypertension may persist even after removal of the primary renal cause (for example, renal artery stenosis) as a result of irreversible damage in the contralateral kidney or structural changes in resistance vessels. Even in mild uncomplicated essential hypertension, there is evidence to suggest that the primary 'lesion' lies in the kidney[1]. There is clearly a wide spectrum of clinical conditions in which renal perfusion, renal function and systemic blood pressure are closely interrelated.

Many surveys have indicated that renal causes account for about 5% of all cases of hypertension[2]. This figure varies according to whether the survey population relates to specialist referral centres, where the prevalence of 'secondary' causes is greater, or to the general population, including milder and 'borderline' hypertension, for which the prevalence is much lower. Even in hypertension that is clearly secondary to a renal disorder, several different mechanisms may contribute.

Chronic renal failure, whatever the cause, may be complicated by hypertension. Here, the principal factor is salt retention and water retention with fluid overload that develops as a result of the loss of renal parenchyma[3]. Glomerulonephritis is the commonest single cause of chronic renal failure[4] but its contribution to hypertension in patients with a normal serum creatinine is less certain, because few such patients undergo renal biopsy. Chronic pyelonephritis is the commonest renal disorder found in the screening of hypertensive patients[2,5] but its relationship with the hypertension is often unclear. Bilateral chronic pyelonephritis causing hypertension is usually accompanied by significant renal impairment. Unilateral disease may also occasionally cause hypertension that may be cured by nephrectomy[6]; in these patients increased renin production by the affected kidney may explain the response to surgery. It is also now apparent that many patients previously classified as having chronic pyelonephritis actually represent cases of interstitial nephritis and/or analgesic nephropathy[7].

In hypertension that is secondary to renal artery stenosis, activation of the renin–angiotensin–aldosterone system undoubtedly contributes to the rise in blood pressure[8], although the mechanisms are much more complex than suggested by the original classical experiment of Goldblatt[9].

A third general mechanism that has emerged relates to an impaired production by the kidney of systemic vasodilator substances such as prostaglandins, kinins and renomedullary lipids. The role of these systems, severally and jointly, and their relationship to drug action, remains speculative.

Any distinction between hypertension that is renal in origin and 'essential' hypertension is important only for a relatively small number of patients in whom a surgical cure is possible. Whatever the underlying cause, uncontrolled hypertension damages the kidneys and effective treatment improves the prognosis.

In a hypertensive population, the renal function at presentation is an important determinant of long-term prognosis. Data from a large multicentre study in the United Kingdom (DHCCP), using a Cox proportional hazards model for analysis, suggest that in hypertension

2

the risk of death increases by 7% for each 1 mmol/l increment in serum urea concentration at presentation[10]. The presence of proteinuria also has an important adverse effect on prognosis.

The early Veterans Administration trials[11,12] showed that drug treatment of severe hypertension was effective in preventing renal failure, although most of the benefit in these studies was accounted for by prevention of accelerated hypertension, stroke and congestive heart failure. The development of renal failure in untreated hypertension was directly related to the severity of the hypertension[13]. With effective treatment, death from renal failure in hypertensive patients is now much less common[14], although progressive nephrosclerosis does occur in a small proportion of treated patients. Renal artery stenosis leading to renal failure may also develop as a *consequence* of long-standing hypertension rather than vice versa (the more traditional view). Data from the eastern United States indicates that 'hypertensive nephropathy' accounts for an increasing proportion of patients entering the Medicare end-stage renal disease (ESRD) programme[15]. In the years 1973–79, hypertensive nephropathy was by far the commonest cause of ESRD in the Black population, the average incidence in Black men being 35 per million person-years compared with 5 per million person-years in White men.

The diagnosis of 'hypertensive nephropathy', as in many other epidemiological studies, suffers from lack of precision. The main difficulty is that ESRD is often characterized by small, shrunken kidneys that may result from chronic renal parenchymal disease, such as glomerulonephritis, pyelonephritis or analgesic nephropathy, or from hypertensive nephrosclerosis. The clinical, radiological and histological features may be indistinguishable at this stage. Nevertheless, recent data from the European Dialysis and Transplantation Association[16,17] also tend to confirm, at least in some European countries, an increasing number of patients accepted for renal replacement therapy whose primary diagnosis is hypertension. Hypertensive disease accounted for 7.2% of 93 037 new patients accepted for renal replacement therapy in Europe between 1976 and 1982. A substantial proportion of these were classified as suffering from renovascular disease secondary to hypertension. There are major international differences in the patterns of acceptance into ESRD programmes even in Europe, but the data indicate a steep increase in the acceptance of patients with hypertension and vascular disease, particularly in the older age groups. The acceptance rate in this category has been increasing approximately in parallel with that in diabetic nephropathy.

The evidence thus suggests that rapidly progressive renal failure due to severe hypertension can be prevented by effective antihypertensive treatment. Untreated hypertension may also result in progressive nephrosclerosis resulting in chronic renal failure. Even with effective therapy, hypertensive patients remain at risk of end-stage failure from nephrosclerosis and from atheromatous renovascular disease and those who reach this stage are now more likely to be candidates for renal replacement therapy.

RENAL HYPERTENSION

This section outlines those renal disorders that are associated with, if not necessarily always the cause of, hypertension (Table 1.1). It includes a brief review of factors that influence decisions about the choice of drug treatment in those conditions.

Renal parenchymal disease

Acute glomerulonephritis

The hypertension in this acute syndrome is usually accompanied by oedema and is closely associated with the phase of oliguria. The hypertension usually resolves as the underlying renal disease remits. In this acute phase, salt and water restriction may be sufficient to control the hypertension. Loop diuretics are often required to control the oedema and will usually reduce the blood pressure at the same time. Supplementary antihypertensive therapy and, occasionally, haemodialysis may be required.

4

TABLE 1.1   Renal disorders associated with hypertension

Renal parenchymal disease

Acute glomerulonephritis
Analgesic nephropathy
Diabetic nephropathy
Chronic glomerulonephritis
Obstructive uropathy
  acute
  chronic (hydronephrosis)
Polycystic kidneys
Pyelonephritis/interstitial nephritis
Unilateral small kidney

Renovascular disease

Renal infarction
Renal artery stenosis
  atheroma
  fibromuscular dysplasia
Arteritis
  polyarteritis nodosa
  systemic lupus erythematosus
  scleroderma
  Takayasu's disease
Trauma
  occlusion/dissection of renal artery
  perirenal haematoma

Analgesic nephropathy

This is a syndrome of middle-aged women who present with hypertension and chronic renal failure[18]. Peptic ulcer and anaemia are also common. The predominant renal lesion is renal papillary necrosis, but chronic interstitial nephritis and transitional cell tumours also occur. Prolonged consumption of any non-steroidal anti-inflammatory drug may be responsible. Proprietary mixtures of aspirin, phenacetin and paracetamol, with or without caffeine, are most frequently implicated, especially when used for headaches. Wide geographical differences exist in the prevalence of this syndrome. It accounts for up to 17% of cases of ESRD requiring renal replacement therapy in Australia[19] and an estimated 7% of all cases of chronic renal disease in the United States[7]. Whether or not the patient discontinues analgesic abuse, hypertension will aggravate the renal impairment and should be controlled.

Diabetic nephropathy

This important complication of long-standing insulin-dependent diabetes is characterized by progressive renal failure and proteinuria and is often accompanied by hypertension. The characteristic histological abnormality is a nodular intercapillary glomerulosclerosis[20]. Renal plasma flow may be increased in the early stages of the disease, but as the disease progresses, widespread hyaline degeneration of glomerular arterioles results in reduced renal perfusion pressure and plasma flow. In this situation, glomerular filtration rate (GFR) is highly sensitive to the influence of the renin-angiotensin system. Efferent arteriolar vasoconstriction by angiotensin II results in glomerular hypertension, increased proteinuria and possibly progression of the glomerulopathy.

Systemic hypertension commonly accompanies diabetic nephropathy and contributes significantly to the progression to end-stage renal failure. Until recently the only form of treatment that had been shown to retard the decline in renal function was early aggressive antihypertensive therapy[21]. Although uncontrolled, this study does provide evidence that treatment of even mild hypertension slows the rate of decline in GFR and the degree of albuminuria in the absence of changes in blood glucose. The principal drug regimen chosen in this study was a 'stepped care' combination of metoprolol, hydralazine and frusemide. Several recent studies have introduced some new therapeutic possibilities. Angiotensin converting enzyme (ACE) inhibitor drugs have been shown to reduce the degree of proteinuria in the absence of a significant effect on blood pressure in hypertensive diabetics with renal failure[22]. Two other studies have shown that in patients with diabetic nephropathy, captopril may reduce the blood pressure, reduce the degree of albuminuria and stabilize or retard the deterioration in glomerular filtration rate[23,24]. It has not yet been clearly established, however, whether these improvements occur independently of the change in systemic blood pressure.

6

It has been suggested as a result of these studies that ACE inhibitors should be considered as drugs of first choice for the treatment of hypertension in diabetic nephropathy. Before this recommendation can be widely adopted, however, some important precautions should be considered. It is as yet uncertain at what stage in the disease such therapy should be introduced or whether ACE inhibitors should be used in the absence of hypertension. Most importantly, it must be borne in mind that hypertension, renal failure and proteinuria are not associated exclusively with glomerulopathy in diabetes. Other renal lesions may coexist that would respond less well or in a different way to therapy with ACE inhibitors. In particular, renal artery stenosis[25] is commonly found in diabetic patients. One must remember that severe bilateral stenoses may be present despite normal levels of serum creatinine, normal intravenous pyelogram and normal isotope renogram. Far from stabilizing or improving renal function, therapy with ACE inhibitors may precipitate or exacerbate renal failure in such patients. If ACE inhibitors are used to treat hypertension in diabetes, it is prudent to undertake full renal investigation prior to initiating therapy and mandatory to monitor renal function during follow-up. Measurement of serum creatinine concentration is inadequate in itself as a means of evaluating baseline renal function, because a significant fall in glomerular filtration rate occurs before the creatinine level rises[26]. Measurement of glomerular filtration rate using ^{51}Cr EDTA or ^{99m}Tc DTPA will provide the most accurate baseline estimate, whereas serum creatinine level may be a simpler and less expensive means of measuring change in renal function in patients with renal impairment. Bilateral renovascular disease should be suspected if renal function worsens. The best way to confirm this diagnosis is by digital subtraction angiography using an intra-arterial injection of contrast.

Some of the attributes of ACE inhibitors and other first- and second-line drugs for controlling hypertension in diabetic patients are summarized in Table 1.2. None of the disadvantages listed in the table are absolute contraindications to their use in diabetes and many combinations of these and other 'third-line' drugs are possible.

There is an urgent need for well-controlled, parallel group comparisons of the several treatment regimens now available, with progression of nephropathy and mortality as the principal end points.

TABLE 1.2   Antihypertensive therapy in diabetic nephropathy

Drug	Advantages	Disadvantages
ACE inhibitors	No adverse effects on: carbohydrate metabolism, lipid metabolism, peripheral blood flow Diminution in proteinuria ?Preservation of renal function	Nephrotoxicity in renovascular disease Renal clearance
β-Adrenoceptor antagonists	Anti-anginal action ??cardioprotection ?preservation of renal function	Peripheral ischaemia Masking of hypoglycaemia Delayed recovery from hypoglycaemia (non-selective drugs only)
Calcium antagonists	No adverse effects on: carbohydrate metabolism, lipid metabolism, peripheral blood flow Antianginal action hepatic clearance	
Hydralazine	No adverse effects on: carbohydrate metabolism, lipid metabolism, peripheral blood flow, renal function	Lupus syndrome Reflex tachycardia

TABLE 1.2 (*contd*)

Drug	Advantages	Disadvantages
Methyldopa	No adverse effects on: carbohydrate metabolism, lipid metabolism, peripheral blood flow, renal function	
Prazosin	No adverse effects on: carbohydrate metabolism, lipid metabolism, peripheral blood flow, renal function	First dose and postural hypo-tension
Thiazide diuretics	No adverse effects on: peripheral blood flow	Hypokalaemia Lipid disturbance Loss of efficacy in severe renal impairment

Chronic glomerulonephritis

This is the commonest cause of ESRD. Hypertension is an accompany-ing feature in over 80% at this stage; it exacerbates the renal damage and adversely affects the cardiovascular system. Hypertension, however, also frequently occurs early in the course of the disease when renal function is still preserved[3]. It may remain asymptomatic at this stage while adversely affecting the kidneys and thus it is important to monitor the blood pressure regularly and treat hypertension in order to preserve renal function. The predominant mechanism is volume overload[3]. There is insufficient evidence on which to judge whether any one antihypertensive regimen is superior in preventing the decline in renal function.

Obstructive uropathy

Acute

Hypertension is a relatively common accompaniment of acute urinary obstruction – either unilateral (e.g. ureteric calculus) or bilateral (e.g. bladder neck obstruction). In the case of bilateral obstruction, reversible acute renal impairment may contribute by causing volume overload. In both bilateral and unilateral obstruction, the rise in blood pressure may be related more to the pain than to the renal dysfunction. This form of hypertension usually regresses with relief of the obstruction and seldom requires antihypertensive therapy. The combination of hypertension and ureteric calculus should stimulate a search for primary hyperparathyroidism. Thiazide diuretics may be useful in the management of idiopathic hypercalciuria with recurrent nephrocalcinosis.

Chronic (hydronephrosis)

Chronic urinary obstruction of any cause may be complicated by hypertension. In bilateral obstruction, the predominant mechanism is volume overload related to the impaired renal function. The hypertension usually resolves if the renal function improves after relief of the obstruction. Unilateral obstruction may occasionally be accompanied by hypertension. This is usually reversible unless permanent hypertensive changes have occurred in the contralateral kidney. Nephrectomy is occasionally indicated for a severely damaged kidney, especially if it is the site of recurrent or persistent infection, and this may also result in cure of the hypertension.

Adult polycystic kidney disease

Blood pressure may be elevated before the serum creatinine level rises[27], and if uncontrolled contributes to the decline in renal function. There is an additional risk of cerebral/subarachnoid haemorrhage in these patients because of an increased prevalence of berry aneurysms[28]. For this reason alone, many clinicians believe that 'target' blood pressures should be set lower in such patients than in other hypertensives. It has yet to be proved that the more aggressive antihypertensive therapy that this entails results in a better outcome in terms of cerebral events or renal function, but every effort should be made to maintain a diastolic blood pressure of less than 90 mmHg. There is no indication that one treatment regimen is superior to another. Recent developments[20] have shown that the gene for this autosomal dominant disorder is located in chromosome 16. This enhances the possibility of early detection and effective genetic counselling of these patients, together with the possibility of earlier diagnosis and antihypertensive therapy that may delay the development of end-stage renal failure.

Pylonephritis/interstitial nephritis

When hypertensive patients are screened by intravenous pyelography, the commonest renal abnormalities detected are those traditionally associated with chronic pyelonephritis[2]. It is now recognized, however, that the common appearances of asymmetrical scarring and calyceal distortion may also occur in analgesic nephropathy. Furthermore, there is good evidence that so-called chronic pyelonephritis is but the end-product of a number of assaults on the kidney, including anatomical abnormalities, obstruction, reflux, stone formation, hyperuricaemia, analgesic abuse and nephrosclerosis[7]. Bacterial infection may complicate the picture in adult life but is seldom the primary cause of the renal scarring and seldom contributes to deterioration in renal function. Most scarring occurs in the first 4 years of life, when reflux nephropathy and recurrent urinary infections combine to damage the kidney. Prevention of recurrent urinary infections is of paramount importance at this stage.

Renin production by the affected kidney in unilateral disease may cause hypertension. In this situation, renal vein renin sampling may reveal an abnormal ratio that favours a successful outcome from nephrectomy. A number of reports suggest that removal of a shrunken, poorly functioning kidney facilitates the control of hypertension[6]. Provided that the disease is unilateral and that the contralateral kidney has not suffered secondary hypertensive nephrosclerosis, the blood pressure will return to normal off treatment or will be easier to control in at least 50% of patients after nephrectomy.

If nephrectomy is not possible, then good control of the blood pressure should be sought in order to preserve renal function. The choice of antihypertensive drug in this context is not critical. Thiazide diuretics may be indicated if there is associated hypercalciuria but should be avoided if there is hyperuricaemia.

Unilateral small kidney

A unilateral small kidney may be congenital or may be the end result of chronic scarring or of renal artery stenosis. It is often impossible to decide what has caused the small kidney and whether or not it is contributing to the hypertension. Removal of a small, poorly functioning kidney should be considered in patients with severe hypertension, but the chances of curing the hypertension will be greater if the function in the contralateral kidney is normal.

Renovascular disease

Renal infarction

Hypertension may develop as a result of infarction of the entire kidney[30] and of major renal embolism secondary to heart disease[31]. However, even segmental renal infarction may result in severe, accelerated hypertension[32].

The need for antihypertensive drug therapy for these patients should be reviewed periodically, as the hypertension may occasionally resolve spontaneously. Similar considerations apply in the management of hypertension associated with acute traumatic occlusion, dissection of the renal artery, or perirenal haematoma.

Renal artery stenosis

There are several reasons why renal artery stenosis (RAS) has remained a most important association with hypertension since the original experiments of Goldblatt and his colleagues[9]. RAS sometimes causes hypertension, and correction of the lesion may restore blood pressure to normal. Hypertension resulting from RAS is often refractory to drug therapy. Much time and effort is therefore spent in the diagnosis and management of this condition. Its greater significance, however, lies in its central role in our understanding of the pathophysiology of hypertension and renal ischaemia, in the application of sophisticated diagnostic techniques, and more recently in the development of antihypertensive drugs, particularly those acting at various sites in the renin–angiotensin–aldosterone system.

The mechanisms underlying the development of hypertension after a stenosing clip has been applied to the renal artery in animals are reasonably well understood[8] and are principally mediated by the release of renin from the affected kidney. The picture in human hypertension is far less clear; two important differences are the time course of the disease and the nature of the stenosing lesion.

The main problem in the time course of human RAS is that if the associated hypertension has been sufficiently severe or prolonged, or both, then arteriolar and glomerular damage may have been inflicted on the contralateral kidney. Even if the stenosis caused the hypertension in the first place, the hypertension may persist after the stenosis is corrected, either because of continuing production of renin or by the loss of renal parenchyma. Other factors contributing to persistent hypertension include structural changes in peripheral resistance vessels and left ventricular hypertrophy. These considerations apply, of course, to any form of 'secondary' hypertension.

Various management regimens, including drug therapy, nephrectomy, autotransplantation, surgical revascularization by a variety of techniques and, more recently, percutaneous transluminal angioplasty (PTA) by balloon catheter have been used in RAS with a view to restoring the blood pressure towards normal or conserving renal function. The continuing search for better means both of diagnosis and of predicting a successful outcome from intervention attests to the less than perfect results from many of these procedures.

The diagnosis of RAS can only be made by arteriography. The development in recent years of techniques of digital subtraction angiography (DSA) has facilitated the investigation of these patients. Acceptable definition can often be achieved using an intravenous injection of contrast medium, but many radiologists still prefer the intra-arterial route for visualizing the renal vessels. Excellent definition can usually be obtained using a low volume of contrast medium, but the technique still carries a small risk, primarily of haematoma formation and arterial injury.

There is much less agreement about the best way to predict the outcome of surgery or PTA. Selective venous sampling for renin is still considered to be useful by some authorities[33], whereas the balance of opinion in the U.K. appears to be that this is merely the best of a number of far-from-perfect predictive tests[34,35]. It is important to remember that renin studies are best undertaken with the patient off drugs. If antihypertensive therapy is considered essential, then prazosin is to be preferred – if only as a temporary measure – as this drug does not significantly interfere with the renin–angiotensin–aldosterone system. The use of drugs intended to stimulate the production of renin, such as diuretics or ACE inhibitors, has not greatly enhanced the predictive power of renin estimations.

The nature of the underlying disease is one important factor relating to the difficulty in predicting outcome. Renal artery stenosis caused by a clip applied to the renal artery of a healthy dog is clearly very different from that associated with the insidious encroachment of an atheromatous plaque in an arteriopathic patient. The two main causes of human RAS are atheroma and fibromuscular dysplasia. Even atheromatous stenosis may take several different forms, each of which may respond very differently to intervention. Ostial stenosis is usually due to extension of a large aortic plaque and is poorly suited to PTA. An isolated stenosis about 1 cm from the origin of the renal artery is often ideally suited to PTA, but the outcome may depend on whether or not the distal arterioles are affected by chronic hypertensive damage. A third pattern, often seen in patients with widespread arteriosclerosis, is that of extensive irregular atheroma extending from the ostium into the renal substance. This pattern is not amenable to PTA and may defy attempted by-pass or reconstruction by even the most skilled vascular surgeon. Clinical and radiological features are therefore often just as important as tests of function in determining outcome.

Fibromuscular dysplasia

This is a condition that predominantly affects young or middle-aged women. The disease is often unilateral and the angiographic appearance is often characteristic. PTA is usually technically successful in these patients and results in cure or amelioration of the hypertension in about 90% of them[36,37]; it is generally thought to be accompanied by excellent long-term survival, although firm data on this are lacking at present. The procedure can be recommended as first-line therapy for all such patients. Antihypertensive drugs may be necessary to control blood pressure pending intervention and as supplementary therapy in the event of an incomplete response to PTA.

Atheroma

Atheromatous lesions in the renal artery are commonly seen in normotensive patients undergoing arteriography for aortic or peripheral vascular disease. The prevalence increases with age[38]. Atheromatous RAS is also commonly found at autopsy in normotensive patients[39]. Bilateral disease is common. The success rate of intervention is much less than in fibromuscular dysplasia[36] and is unpredictable.

Many studies on this subject have focused on aspects of diagnosis, techniques of intervention and clinical responses in respect of blood pressure and renal function. The observation of a high mortality in such patients, irrespective of intervention, is of equal importance. The 4-year mortality in patients identified as having renal artery stenosis in the Glasgow Blood Pressure Clinic exceeds 30%[40]. This high mortality reflects the widespread atheromatous disease in many of these patients, affecting not only the renal arteries but also the coronary and cerebral vessels. PTA is still possible, though technically more difficult, especially in patients with severe aortic disease and ostial stenosis[41]. Observational studies indicate that progression of disease, often to complete occlusion, occurs in about half of such patients observed over a 3-year period[42], and there is some evidence[43], albeit from uncontrolled studies, that surgical intervention improves the prognosis. The results from surgery or angioplasty in specialist centres are certainly impressive, even in patients with renal failure[44] and in cases of totally occluded renal arteries[45], but we lack a direct comparison of medical therapy versus intervention in a concurrent, randomized study.

There is a particular need to compare both surgery and PTA with a primary medical regimen in older patients, those with bilateral disease, severe aortic disease and renal impairment. The study endpoints should include mortality and quality-of-life assessments.

One of the explanations for the inferior response to intervention in RAS due to atheroma compared with that due to fibromuscular dysplasia is that atheromatous disease of the renal arteries may develop *as a result of*, or coincidentally with, long-standing essential hypertension. It is just as likely that hypertension, cigarette-smoking, diabetes and hyperlipidaemias predispose to atheromatous renal artery disease as they do to disease in the coronary, cerebral and peripheral arteries.

Antihypertensive drug therapy

Drug therapy is often required in patients with RAS for whom operative intervention is not possible or in whom the hypertension persists after surgery or PTA, or as a short-term measure while patients undergo investigation and await surgery. It is important in these circumstances that treatment should not adversely affect renal function[46]. Excessive or precipitous hypotension must be avoided as renal failure may result from reduced perfusion or even from renal artery thrombosis or occlusion. This is probably a general risk, attributable as much to the magnitude of the fall in blood pressure as to any more specific pharmacological effect. Renal artery occlusion has been reported after treatment with β-adrenoceptor antagonists[47] and with ACE inhibitors[48] although it is very difficult to know whether occlusion was due to the antihypertensive drugs or simply the usual progression of the underlying disease.

ACE inhibitors may, however, pose additional and more specific adverse pharmacological effects in renal artery stenosis. Several reports now attest to the risk of renal failure when such drugs are used for renovascular hypertension[49,50]. The risks are greatest in patients with bilateral disease (Figure 1.1) or stenosis in a solitary or transplanted kidney. Even in unilateral RAS, ACE inhibitors frequently cause severe deterioration of glomerular filtration rate in the affected kidney[51], although detection of this problem requires split renal function tests. The problem may be caused by blockade of angiotensin II formation and the resultant reduction in efferent renal arteriolar tone. Glomerular filtration rate may be adversely affected *without* a large drop in systemic arterial pressure or in renal blood flow. The deterioration in renal function may be insidious, developing over several months, but is usually at least partly reversible. Since ACE inhibitors and their active metabolites are eliminated by the kidney, they accumulate as renal function declines, resulting in a 'vicious spiral' of falling

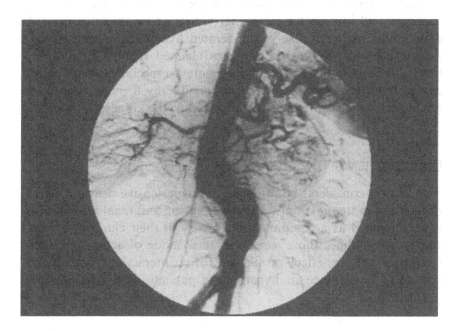

FIGURE 1.1   Digital subtraction aortogram in a 70-year-old patient, showing a severely atheromatous aorta and bilateral renal artery stenosis. This patient's serum creatinine rose from 126 μmol/l to 737 μmol/l over a period of 6 months after the institution of therapy with enalapril 5 mg once daily and bendrofluazide 5 mg once daily for severe hypertension. Cessation of ACE inhibitor therapy was followed by an improvement in serum creatinine. (Reproduced by courtesy of Dr R.G. Mahaffey.)

17

blood pressure and rising creatinine levels. All patients exhibiting a deterioration in renal function on ACE inhibitors require investigation to identify the nature of the underlying renal disease. ACE inhibitors must be used at minimal dosage with the greatest caution and only with careful monitoring of renal function in patients with renovascular hypertension.

Arteritis

Takayasu's disease is recognized as a cause of secondary hypertension in Asiatics[52] but is notably rare in Western populations. Polyarteritis nodosa, progressive systemic sclerosis and systemic lupus erythematosus may all involve the intrarenal vessels and may be associated with a fulminating course of accelerated hypertension and rapidly progressive renal failure. It has been claimed that ACE inhibitor therapy is of particular benefit in this context, especially in renal crises caused by scleroderma[53,54], but occasionally any form of aggressive antihypertensive therapy may help to salvage the kidneys.

DRUGS IN RENAL HYPERTENSION AND RENAL FAILURE

This section considers the principal antihypertensive drugs in terms of their use in treatment of renal hypertension and renal failure. This is not intended as a comprehensive review of their clinical pharmacology but outlines those aspects of their mode of action, pharmacokinetics, adverse-effect profile and drug interactions that are of particular importance in hypertensive patients with renal disease (Table 1.3).

Adrenergic neurone-blocking drugs

Drugs in this category, such as bethanidine, debrisoquine and guanethidine are generally reserved as third-line agents because of their troublesome adverse effects of postural and exercise hypotension, diarrhoea, fluid retention and sexual dysfunction in men. However,

TABLE 1.3 Antihypertensive drugs and renal hypertension

Drug	Problems in renal hypertension	Dosage adjustments in renal failure
Adrenergic neurone blocking drugs		reduce (avoid guanethidine)
ACE inhibitors	renal failure (RAS) proteinuria } especially in neutropenia scleroderma, P. nodosa, SLE	reduce
Calcium antagonists	—	—
β-Adrenoceptor antagonists	minimal rise in creatinine ?? renal artery thrombosis	reduce (atenolol) no change (metoprolol) ?(propranolol)
Diazoxide	precipitous hypotension, azotaemia	reduce
Diuretics thiazide	hypokalaemia, hyperuricaemia rise in urea, creatinine	loss of efficacy
loop	hypokalaemia, hyperuricaemia rise in urea, creatinine	increase
K-sparing	hyperkalaemia	avoid
Glyceryl trinitrate	—	—
Hydralazine	??risk of lupus	do not exceed 100 mg/day
Methyldopa	Excessive hypotension	reduce
Minoxidil	Fluid retention	reduce
Nitroprusside	Cyanide toxicity	reduce
Prazosin	Excessive hypotension Neuropsychiatric effects	reduce

they have no direct nephrotoxic effects and are still occasionally useful in patients with renal hypertension who are intolerant of other drugs.

Guanethidine is poorly and variably absorbed after oral administration, its clearance is predominantly renal, but its elimination half life of 3–5 days reflects tissue binding. It should be avoided in renal failure because of the risk of accumulation and possible aggravation of oedema. Bethanidine is also excreted mainly by the kidneys and, although it is a shorter-acting drug than guanethidine, accumulation may also lead to problems in renal failure. Debrisoquine undergoes polymorphic hydroxylation in the liver: approximately 10% of subjects are poor hydroxylators and are more susceptible to adverse effects at a given dosage. Debrisoquine, however, will also accumulate in severe renal impairment and dosage should be reduced.

Angiotensin converting enzyme (ACE) inhibitors

The two principal drugs in this group are captopril[55] and enalapril[56]. Several others are at an advanced stage of development. The principal action of these drugs is blockade of angiotensin II synthesis by inhibition of the converting enzyme peptidyldipeptide hydrolase. The same enzyme also degrades bradykinin, accumulation of which may also contribute to the fall in blood pressure. There is evidence to show that the antihypertensive effect of ACE inhibitors is greater after the renin–angiotensin system has been stimulated by salt and water depletion[57]. On the other hand, captopril reduces the blood pressure in fluid-depleted patients with very low plasma concentrations of active renin[58]; this suggests that circulating levels of renin in plasma do not directly determine the action of ACE inhibitors. The explanation may be that these drugs act directly on the renin system known to be present in the vessel wall[59].

Captopril was initially used at doses up to 450 mg daily in patients with severe hypertension, often with pre-existing renal disease. Numerous reports appeared describing the development of adverse effects in these patients including proteinuria, skin rashes, loss of taste and neutropenia[60]. These were attributed in part to the presence of a sulphydryl group in the captopril molecule, but it subsequently became apparent that dosage and patient factors were equally important contributors to the problem of toxicity. Many of the patients with significant proteinuria on captopril had pre-existing renal disease and the vast majority of patients who developed agranulocytosis had serious underlying medical disorders and were on multiple concurrent drug therapy. The use of lower doses of captopril, especially in patients with renal impairment and connective tissue disorders, has resulted in an improved safety profile[61,62].

Enalapril was introduced at much lower doses, initially as mono-therapy in patients with mild, uncomplicated hypertension, and its use was only later extended to the management of more severe, com-plicated or secondary hypertension. As a result, its adverse effects profile is reassuring[63].

Haematological problems are now very rare with both drugs. Skin rashes and taste disturbances are uncommon but may be marginally more frequent on captopril. Coughing and proteinuria are also uncom-mon. However, hypotension and renal failure remain significant prob-lems with both drugs.

Both ACE inhibitors may cause potentially serious first-dose hypo-tension[64,65]. The risk is greatest in patients that are sodium-depleted, usually as a result of concurrent diuretic therapy, although relatively modest doses of thiazide may predispose to this problem[66]. Patients with severe, complicated or renovascular hypertension[64] and patients with cardiac failure[67] may also be at increased risk. The predominant features of first-dose hypotension in hypertensive patients are focal neurological signs; syncope and renal impairment predominate in heart failure. The hypotension is usually accompanied by bradycardia, reflecting the parasympathomimetic effect of ACE inhibitors[67].

In the context of renal hypertension, the other common serious adverse effect of ACE inhibitors is renal failure. This is especially likely to occur in hypertensive patients with bilateral RAS[49] (see also Figure 1.1), with unilateral RAS and a contralateral non-functioning kidney, or with RAS in a transplanted kidney[68]. Concomitant diuretic therapy may increase the risk[50]. Deterioration in renal function in an affected kidney may be observed after a single oral dose of captopril[69] or may develop gradually over several months. Detection of loss of function in a kidney affected by unilateral RAS may require the use of split renal function tests[51]. The impairment of renal function is usually reversible, at least in the first few weeks, although in some cases thrombotic occlusion of the renal artery is an additional hazard[48]. The deterioration in renal function may occur without a large drop in systemic blood pressure and the mechanism is thought to relate to loss of influence of angiotensin II on the renal efferent arteriole with a resultant reduction in filtration pressure. This is especially likely to occur when the perfusion pressure to the kidney is reduced by severe arterial disease or by cardiac failure.

Both captopril and enalaprilat (the active metabolite of enalapril) are eliminated via the kidney. The dosage must be reduced in renal failure. ACE inhibition should be used only with the greatest caution if there is any suspicion of renal impairment, and it should be mandatory to monitor renal function. A rise in the serum creatinine during the course of treatment with ACE inhibitors is an indication to investigate the possibility of renovascular disease[70].

The major use of ACE inhibitors is likely to be in mild-to-moderate essential hypertension, when their effect on blood pressure is approximately similar to that of β-adrenoceptor antagonists and when they can usefully be combined with low-dose diuretic therapy[71,72]. Their relative lack of symptomatic adverse effects may be an advantage[73] although there is a lack of data relating to their long-term effects on morbidity and mortality.

The possible advantages of therapy with ACE inhibition in diabetic nephropathy have been discussed earlier in this chapter. ACE inhibitors are undoubtedly effective in the treatment of renovascular hypertension[74], but their efficacy in lowering blood pressure must be tempered by their adverse effects on renal function in affected kidneys. ACE inhibitors are also possibly of particular value in scleroderma renal crises[54], but controlled studies are clearly difficult in that condition and interpretation of reported cases can be uncertain. In general, ACE inhibitors should be used with the greatest caution in any form of pre-existing renal disease.

The safest, most effective, way to use ACE inhibitor therapy in hypertension is to start with monotherapy at low doses (captopril 12.5 mg, enalapril 2.5 mg). It is seldom profitable to increase the dosage of captopril above 50 mg three times a day or of enalapril above 20 mg once daily. If these doses fail to control the blood pressure, a thiazide diuretic should be added in low dosage and, failing that, a loop diuretic. It has yet to be shown whether it is better to adopt a policy of increasing the dose of loop diuretics or of adding a third or fourth drug such as a β-adrenoceptor antagonist, calcium antagonist or other vasodilator. ACE inhibitors have not solved the problem of refractory hypertension or the need for polypharmacy in many patients.

Beta-adrenoceptor antagonists

Propranolol reduces both renal blood flow[75] and glomerular filtration rate[76] in hypertensive patients with normal renal function although these changes are not of clinical significance. Even in hypertensive patients with mild renal impairment, propranolol does not cause deterioration in renal function[77]. On a more cautionary note, however, deterioration in renal function has been reported after the use of β-adrenoceptor antagonists in patients with moderately severe chronic renal failure[78]. Renal impairment became apparent within a few weeks of introducing propranolol and oxprenolol but has also been reported after a single dose of atenolol[47]. The mechanism probably relates to a fall in renal perfusion pressure resulting from the reduction in cardiac output, although renal artery thrombosis may supervene, particularly in patients with severe atheroma.

The influence of ancillary properties of β-adrenoceptor antagonists on renal function – such as cardioselectivity, partial agonist activity and membrane-stabilizing activity – has not been established. It now seems clear that the antihypertensive action of these drugs is mediated through β1 rather than β2 adrenoceptors[79]. Vasodilator effects of catecholamines, including those in peripheral and renal arteries, are mediated principally by β2 effects. There are sound theoretical reasons for preferring a drug that selectively blocks β1 receptors, minimizing the unnecessary blockade of β2 receptors with the resultant adverse effects of obstruction of airways, vasoconstriction and impaired gluconeogenesis. In treating hypertension in diabetic patients, with or without nephropathy, cardioselective drugs such as atenolol or metoprolol are definitely to be preferred because they are less likely to delay the recovery from hypoglycaemia[80,81]. In other forms of renal hypertension, however, it must be admitted that differences between β-adrenoceptor antagonists with different pharmacodynamic properties may be of marginal clinical importance.

23

β-Adrenoceptor antagonists are widely used in all forms of hypertension. Many studies have confirmed that the dose–response curve of these drugs is relatively flat and that a reduction in blood pressure of up to 20/15 mmHg can be achieved with monotherapy[82]. The effects on blood pressure of the combination of β-adrenoceptor antagonists with other drugs such as diuretics, vasodilators or methyldopa are at least additive. Contrary to what is widely perceived, the onset of antihypertensive effect of β-adrenoceptor antagonists is rapid (within a few hours of oral administration[83]) and this property can be useful in the prompt control even of accelerated hypertension[84].

Many β-adrenoceptor antagonists are now available, all differing in their pharmacodynamic and pharmacokinetic properties. These have been expertly reviewed elsewhere[85] and are not discussed here in detail. Propranolol undergoes extensive first-pass metabolism in the liver. Its principal metabolite, 4-hydroxypropranolol, has similar β-blocking activity and undergoes glucuronidation before excretion by the kidney. The elimination of propranolol metabolites may be greatly impaired in renal failure[86]. Metoprolol also undergoes extensive hepatic metabolism but its metabolites are inactive[87]. Dosage adjustment in renal failure is not usually necessary, and since metoprolol is also cardioselective it is preferable to propranolol. Atenolol is eliminated almost entirely unchanged by the kidney. It will accumulate in renal failure if usual doses are given but at least there is no uncertainty about active metabolites and it is usually a simple matter to make dose adjustments according to the clinical response.

Calcium antagonists

The principal drug in this group used for hypertension is nifedipine[88]. Nicardipine[89] is a very similar drug that has recently been introduced in the United Kingdom. Verapamil is also a useful antihypertensive. Many others are currently under investigation. These drugs appear to be relatively free of serious toxicity, but their vasodilator properties are poorly tolerated by a substantial proportion of patients. Nifedipine and nicardipine cause facial flushing, headache, palpitations and leg oedema. These problems are dose-related and may relate to saturation of hepatic first-pass metabolism. Verapamil is less prone to these vascular adverse effects but causes constipation and interacts adversely with β-adrenoceptor antagonists and with digoxin.

Nifedipine and nicardipine, as with other dihydropyridines, undergo almost complete hepatic metabolism prior to urinary excretion. Renal failure has little effect on the pharmacokinetics of either drug and dosage modification is unnecessary. Two of the disadvantages of currently available calcium antagonists are, first, the need for individual dose titration and, second, their short duration of action and the consequent need for dosing twice or three times daily to maintain their antihypertensive effect. Amlodipine, currently showing promise in phase 2 studies, may be the first calcium antagonist with genuine once-daily efficacy in hypertension.

Nifedipine and nicardipine are not considered to have adverse effects on renal blood flow or on glomerular filtration rate in patients with normal renal function. Furthermore, both drugs[88,89] have been shown to have diuretic and natriuretic actions that are possibly due to an effect on proximal tubular function. These features, together with the drugs' lack of nephrotoxicity and their pharmacokinetic profiles, would suggest that they might be of value in renal hypertension or hypertension complicated by renal failure. They are indeed widely used in these circumstances, both as first-line and as supplementary therapy, although there is a lack of controlled clinical trials on which to base a judgement of their place in therapy. Nifedipine has been reported to have precipitated acute renal failure in four patients with chronic renal disease, possibly as a result of autoregulatory failure[90], and it would be prudent to use this drug with caution in those circumstances.

Diazoxide

This thiazide-related drug exhibits a direct relaxant effect on resistance vessels. Its powerful antihypertensive effect is accompanied by fluid retention and reflex tachycardia. Intravenous diazoxide was widely used in the past in the treatment of hypertensive emergencies. It was claimed that diazoxide must be administered by rapid bolus injection to be fully effective in accelerated hypertension[91]. However, when used in this way, its hypertensive action is sudden, unpredictable and

25

difficult to titrate or reverse. As a result patients are put at risk of ischaemic stroke, myocardial infarction and acute renal failure. These problems may, of course, result from precipitous hypotension whichever drug is used. The risk is especially high in accelerated hypertension, when autoregulation of cerebral blood flow is impaired[92]. A more gradual reduction in blood pressure has been reported after slow intravenous infusion of diazoxide[93]. However, with the advent of alternative drugs, there is now little place for the use of diazoxide in modern therapeutics.

Diazoxide is highly bound (over 90%) to albumin. A rapid bolus injection ensures maximal delivery of free drug to resistance vessels and determines the rapidity of response. Protein binding of diazoxide is decreased in renal failure[94] and the resultant increase in free fraction is accompanied by a greater pharmacological effect. In addition, since glomerular filtration accounts for a significant part of the clearance of diazoxide[95], the elimination of the drug will be impaired in renal failure.

Diuretics

Thiazides

During the first few days of therapy with thiazides for hypertension, urine volume and sodium excretion increase and plasma volume declines. With continued therapy for a few weeks, the plasma volume returns towards normal owing, in part, to activation of the renin–angiotensin–aldosterone system. At this stage, the antihypertensive action of long-term thiazide treatment is characterized by a reduction in total peripheral resistance and diminished sensitivity to vasoconstrictor agents. Whether these effects result from changes in electrolyte balance, prostaglandin metabolism or direct vascular effects remains uncertain. Thiazides do not lower the blood pressure in anephric subjects[96] and their antihypertensive effect can be reversed by infusion of saline[97] or co-administration of non-steroidal antiflammatory drugs[98]. These studies suggest that some degree of sodium depletion seems important for their long-term effect, although another study[99] in patients with chronic renal failure raises the possibility of a mechanism independent of sodium loss. Diuretics potentiate most other antihypertensive drugs.

High doses of thiazide diuretics are often accompanied by a rise in plasma urea and creatinine but, at the lower doses required for an antihypertensive action, impairment of renal function is uncommon. The hypokalaemia or hyperuricaemia that occasionally accompanies long-term diuretic therapy may cause renal tubular damage. Diuretics enhance the nephrotoxicity of non-steroidal anti-inflammatory drugs and of ACE inhibitors.

Loop diuretics

Loop diuretics are less effective than thiazides in essential hypertension[100] and their rather short action may also be a disadvantage. However, they are more effective than thiazides in the presence of renal impairment[101] and should generally be substituted when the serum creatinine exceeds 150 μmol/l (this corresponds very approximately with a fall in GFR of about 60%). Loop diuretics have a much steeper dose–response pattern than thiazides (hence the term 'high-ceiling' diuretic) and it may be necessary to use very high doses in advanced renal impairment. This attribute may also be useful in combination therapy with ACE inhibition, when increasing the dose of loop diuretic enhances the antihypertensive effect. This regimen, however, may also predispose to renal failure and must be used with caution.

Potassium-sparing diuretics

Spironolactone, triamterene and amiloride may be useful in hypertensive patients with hypokalaemia secondary to diuretic therapy, but should be avoided in patients with impaired renal function because of the risks of hyperkalaemia, drug accumulation and aggravation of nephrotoxicity.

Glyceryl trinitrate

Most clinicians are aware that glyceryl trinitrate acts as a dilator of coronary arteries and venous capacitance vessels, and as such it finds a use in the treatment of angina pectoris and left ventricular failure. However, it is perhaps less widely appreciated that glyceryl trinitrate at higher doses dilates both resistance arterioles and veins[102]. Variable absorption and rapid metabolism preclude the use of oral dosage, and sublingual and percutaneous routes are more suited to low-dose administration.

Glyceryl trinitrate has a dose-related antihypertensive effect when given by continuous intravenous infusion. The onset and offset are rapid (within minutes) and this facilitates rapid titration of dose against effect. Infusion may be continued for days or weeks if necessary. Glyceryl trinitrate infusion may be accompanied by an increase in heart rate, whereas myocardial oxygen consumption may decrease. Vasodilator headache may occur.

Glyceryl trinitrate is rapidly metabolized in the liver and red blood cells to less active dinitrates, mononitrates and nitrites. The elimination half-life of glyceryl trinitrate is approximately 3 minutes. Kinetic studies in patients with renal failure have not been reported, but no significant changes should be anticipated.

Because of its ease of administration, generally favourable effects on left ventricular function and coronary blood flow, lack of serious metabolic effects, lack of adverse renal effects, and pharmacokinetic properties, glyceryl trinitrate is increasingly used in hypertensive emergencies (including renal hypertension) such as dissecting aneurysm and acute left ventricular failure and to control the blood pressure during and after open-heart surgery.

Hydralazine

Two factors have resulted in a decline in the use of hydralazine as a second-line antihypertensive drug in recent years. One is the increasing use of ACE inhibitors and calcium antagonists. The second is the recognition that even modest doses of hydralazine may result in a lupus syndrome[103]. Nevertheless, hydralazine emerged as the preferred

third drug used to supplement therapy with bendrofluazide plus atenolol in a recent trial reported from Glasgow[104]. Nifedipine and ACE
inhibitors were not included in that study, however, and the results of
further 'third drug' trials are awaited with interest.

Hydralazine does not have adverse effects on the kidney and may
even increase renal blood flow, although GFR does not change. It is
therefore still widely used in both essential and renal hypertension.
The use of hydralazine usually requires the concomitant use of a β-
adrenoceptor antagonist to inhibit reflex tachycardia and a diuretic
to control fluid retention.

Hydralazine is metabolized in the liver, to an extent depending
on the patient's acetylator phenotype. The metabolic pathways of
hydralazine are complex and little is known about the relative con-
tributions of the parent drug or its metabolites to either its hypotensive
or adverse effects. The hydralazine lupus syndrome is more frequent
in women and when the daily dosage exceeds 150 mg and it seldom
occurs other than in slow acetylators. It is now recommended that the
maximum daily dosage of hydralazine should not exceed 100 mg in
men and 50 mg in women[103]. Both the renal clearance and the hepatic
metabolism of hydralazine may be impaired in renal failure[105].

Intravenous hydralazine is a useful drug for short-term intravenous
use to suppress surges in blood pressure, for example during
pregnancy, during operative procedures and in severe hypertension,
although close control of the blood pressure is not possible and
alternative drugs are available for finer tuning of blood pressure.

Methyldopa

Although no longer considered a first-line drug for hypertension,
methyldopa is still one of the most commonly prescribed antihypertensives. At equipotent antihypertensive doses, methyldopa
causes more side-effects than atenolol[106] and is less acceptable than
either prazosin or hydralazine[104]. Despite its large number of adverse
effects, it has not been implicated in renal toxicity, and for this reason
is frequently used in hypertensive patients with renal disease.

The clearance of methyldopa is predominantly renal[107], however,
and dosage should be adjusted accordingly in patients with renal

impairment. It is likely that once-daily administration is sufficient in patients with elevated serum creatinine. If dosage is not adjusted, the main predictable adverse effects are central nervous symptoms and excessive hypotension. Profound 'first-dose' hypotension may occur after methyldopa. Renal failure may result from reduced renal perfusion pressure.

Minoxidil

This direct-acting arteriolar dilator is reserved for the treatment of severe hypertension that is refractory to other drugs[108,109]. It is invariably necessary to use β-adreneceptor antagonists to control the reflex tachycardia that accompanies its use, and loop diuretics, often in large doses, to control the severe peripheral oedema that otherwise develops, particularly in patients with renal impairment. Minoxidil and its glucuronic acid conjugate are excreted by the kidneys[110]. In practice, minoxidil is seldom used in patients with normal renal function and little will be lost by starting with a dose of 2.5 mg once daily and increasing at no more than weekly intervals by 2.5 mg increments. Minoxidil is a potent drug and the use of this cautious regimen will usually avoid excessive hypotension that may occasionally result in renal impairment. Excessive growth of facial hair precludes its use in women.

Sodium nitroprusside

This drug is a powerful dilator of both arteries and veins and as such tends to have a generally beneficial effect on haemodynamics, particularly in patients with left ventricular failure[111]. Intravenous infusion is necessary and results in the onset of effects within a few minutes. The hypotensive effect wears off equally quickly when the infusion is discontinued, thus allowing rapid titration of dose against response. The infusate must be protected from light.

The principal metabolite is cyanide, which is metabolized by the liver to thiocyanate, which is in turn eliminated by renal excretion. Accumulation of cyanide may result in metabolic acidosis and neuropsychiatric toxicity. Thiocyanate inhibits both the uptake and binding of iodide and hypothyroidism has been reported. The infusion rate should not exceed $10 \,\mu\text{g kg}^{-1}\text{min}^{-1}$ and the total dose should not exceed 1.5 mg/kg. The ability to detoxify cyanide may be impaired in liver disease. Elevated thiocyanate levels have been reported in patients with severe renal impairment[111].

Nitroprusside is undoubtedly effective and seldom fails to lower blood blood pressure. It retains an important role in the maintenance of controlled hypotension during anaesthesia – especially for neuro-surgical procedures and during removal of phaeochromocytoma. It has been used successfully in the control of drug-resistant renovascular hypertension[112]. In renal hypertension or in renal impairment, however, it may be best considered a drug of ultimate reserve, because of its potential toxicity.

Prazosin

Prazosin acts as a peripheral competitive α-adrenoceptor antagonist[113] and reduces total peripheral resistance without the reflex tachycardia that commonly accompanies the use of other arteriolar dilators. This may reflect its action on venous capacitance vessels as well as arterioles[114], but this in turn predisposes to postural hypotension that may persist even during long-term therapy. Reports of symptomatic 'first-dose' hypotension[115] discouraged many clinicians from adopting prazosin as a first-line antihypertensive drug. Revised recommendations for dose titration have minimized this problem and some of the advantages of this drug are now more widely appreciated[113].

Prazosin does not have adverse effects on carbohydrate metabolism, renal function, airways calibre, ventricular function or peripheral blood flow. It may have beneficial effects of plasma lipids[116]. It is therefore a useful antihypertensive in renovascular hypertension, in diabetic nephropathy and in renal parenchymal disease.

Prazosin normally undergoes extensive 'first-pass' metabolism in the liver and predominantly biliary excretion. However, its duration of action is prolonged in renal failure[117]. If maintenance dosage in renal failure is not reduced, the usual adverse effects will be exaggerated and, as recently reported[118], additional neuropsychiatric complications may develop.

ANTIHYPERTENSIVE THERAPY IN DIALYSIS PATIENTS

A very small number of patients with ESRD have severe hypertension that remains refractory to 'medical' management in the form of dialysis and multiple drug therapy; these patients may benefit from bilateral nephrectomy. However, the hypertension that accompanies most forms of end-stage renal disease is volume-dependent and responds to removal of salt and water either by haemodialysis or by continuous ambulatory peritoneal dialysis (CAPD). Nevertheless, additional antihypertensive therapy is often required.

Removal of fluid by dialysis results in a fall in blood pressure and additionally potentiates the action of most antihypertensive drugs. This may result in some patients in symptomatic hypotension after dialysis. This problem is unpredictable and may occur with any antihypertensive drug or combination. If the hypotension is severe and persistent, it may be necessary to reduce the frequency of dosing and to omit the antihypertensive therapy prior to dialysis. Some patients show an extreme lability of blood pressure on dialysis, even in the absence of antihypertensive drug therapy.

A second general problem is that some antihypertensive drugs are removed by dialysis. The factors influencing drug pharmacokinetics during dialysis are complex[119] and include molecular size, lipid solubility, protein binding, metabolism and flow rates within the system. The most important single factor, however, is the apparent volume of distribution of the drug and its active metabolites, or, in other words, the degree of binding to tissues and plasma proteins. Generally drugs that are not extensively bound, that are water-soluble, and that are normally eliminated by glomerular filtration will be removed to a significant extent by dialysis. Antihypertensive drugs in this category include atenolol, sotalol and methyldopa. Theoretically, removal of these drugs during dialysis may minimize the risk of post-dialysis hypotension and might even necessitate supplementary dosage to maintain their effect. In practice, it has not been established that this is a major advantage, possibly because the antihypertensive effect of these drugs is not clearly related to their plasma concentrations. The only other major group of dialysable antihypertensive drugs are the ACE inhibitors. Despite the rather efficient removal of these drugs by dialysis, however, their effects are so potentiated by fluid depletion, even in anephric patients, that a reduction in dosage is usually necessary to avoid excessive post-dialysis hypotension[58,120].

References

1. de Wardener, H.E. and MacGregor, G.A. (1982). The natriuretic hormone and essential hypertension. *Lancet* 1, 1450–54
2. Rudnick, K.V., Sackett, D.L., Hirst, S. and Holmes, C. (1977). Hypertension in a family practice. *Can. Med. Assoc. J.*, 117, 492–7
3. Danielsen, H., Kornerup, H.J., Olsen, S.O. and Posburg, V. (1983). Arterial hypertension in chronic glomerulonephritis. An analysis of 310 cases. *Clin. Nephrol.* 19, 284–7
4. Walker, G.G., Bender, W.L. (1984). Management of end-stage renal disease. In Harvey A.McG, Johns, R.J., McKusick, V.A., Owens, A.H., Ross, R.S. *The Principles and Practice of Medicine*, pp 136–148. Connecticut: Appleton-Century-Crofts
5. Dollery, C.T., Beilin, L.J., Bulpitt, C.J., Coles, E.C., Johnson, B.F., Munro-Faure, A.D., Turner, S.C. (1977) Initial care of hypertensive patients. Influence of different types of clinical records. *Br. Heart J.* 39, 181–5
6. Siamopoulos, K., Sellars, L., Mishra, S.C., Essenhigh, D.M., Robson, V., Wilkinson, R. (1983). Experience in the management of hypertension with unilateral chronic pylonephritis: results in nephrectomy in selected patients. *Q. J. Med.* 207, 349–62
7. Murray, T., Goldberg, M. (1975). Chronic interstitial nephritis: etiologic factors. *Ann. Intern. Med.* 82, 453–9
8. Robertson, J.I.S., Morton J.J., Tillman, D.M., Lever, A.F. (1986). The pathophysiology of renovascular hypertension. *J. Hypertension* 4, (Suppl. 4), S95–S103
9. Goldblatt, H., Lynch, R.F., Hanzai, R.F., Summerville, W. (1934). Studies on experimental hypertension, production of persistent elevation of systolic blood pressure by means of renal ischaemia. *J. Exp. Med.* 59, 347–79
10. Bulpitt, C.J., Beevers, D.G., Butler, A., Coles, E.C., Hunt, D., Munro-Faure, A.D., Newson, R.B., O'Riordan, P.W., Petrie, J.C., Rajagopalan, B., Rylance, P.B., Twallin, G., Webster, J., Dollery, C.T. (1986). The survival of treated hypertensive patients and their causes of death: a report from the DHSS hypertensive care computing project (DHCCP). *J. Hypertension* 4, 93–9
11. Veterans Administration Cooperative Study Group on Antihypertensive Agents, Effects of treatment on morbidity in hypertension – results in patients with diastolic blood pressures averaging 115 through 129 mmHg. (1970). *J. Am. Med. Assoc.* 213, 1143–52
12. Veterans Administration Cooperative Study Group on Antihypertensive

Agents, Effects of treatment on morbidity in Hypertension. *ii*. Results in patients with diastolic blood pressure averaging 90 through 114 mmHg. (1970). *J. Am. Med. Assoc.* **213**, 1143–52

13. Smith, D.E., Odel, H.M. and Kernohan, J.W. (1950). Causes of death in hypertension. *Am. J. Med.* **9**, 516–27

14. Bulpitt, C.J., Breckenridge, A. (1976). Plasma urea in hypertensive patients. *Br. Heart J.* **38**, 689–94

15. Sugimoto, T., Rosansky, S.J. (1984). The incidence of treated end stage renal disease in the Eastern United States: 1973–79. *Am. J. Public Health* **74**, 14–17

16. Wing, A.J., Broyer, M., Brunner, F.P., Challah, S., Donckerwolke, R.A., Gretz, N., Jacobs, C., Kramer, P., Selwood, N.H. (1983). Combined report on regular dialysis and transplantation in Europe, XII 1982. *Proc. Eur. Dialy. Transplant. Assoc. – Eur. Renal Assoc.* **20**, 5–75

17. Brunner, F.P., Broyer, M., Brynger, H., Challah, S., Fassbinder, W., Oules, R., Rizzoni, G., Selwood, N.H., Wing, A.J. (1985). Combined report on regular dialysis and transplantation in Europe, XV 1984. *Proc. Eur. Dialy. Transplant. Assoc. – Eur. Renal Assoc.* **22**, 5–53

18. Nanra, R.S. Drug-induced renal disease (1986). *Med. Int. 2nd Series* **33**, 1366–76

19. Shiel, A., Stewart, J., Johnson, J. (1969). Community treatment of end-stage renal failure by dialysis and transplantation from cadaver donors. *Lancet* **2**, 917–20

20. Kimmelstiel, P., Wilson, C. (1936). Intercapillary lesions in the glomeruli of the kidney. *Am. J. Pathol.* **12**, 83–97

21. Parving, H-H., Andersen, A.R., Smidt, U.M., Svendsen, P.A. (1983). Early aggressive antihypertensive treatment reduces rate of decline in kidney function in diabetic nephropathy. *Lancet* **1**, 1175–8

22. Taguma, Y., Kitamoto, Y., Futaki, G., Ueda, H., Monma, H., Ishizaki, M., Takahashi, H., Sekino, H., Sasaki, Y. (1985). Effect of captopril on heavy proteinuria in azotemic diabetics. *N. Engl. J. Med.* **313**, 1617–20

23. Hommel, E., Parving, H.H., Mathiesen, E., Edsberg, B., Nielsen, M.D., Giese, J. (1986). Effect of captopril on kidney function in insulin-dependent diabetic patients with nephropathy. *Br. Med. J.* **293**, 467–70

24. Bjorck, S., Nyberg, G., Mulec, H., Granerus, G., Herlitz, H., Aurell, M. (1986). Beneficial effects of angiotensin converting enzyme inhibitors on renal function in patients with diabetic nephropathy. *Br. Med. J.* **293**, 471–4

25. Shapiro, A.P., Perez-Stable, E., Moutsos, S.E. (1965). Coexistence of renal arterial hypertension and diabetes mellitus. *J. Am. Med. Assoc.* **192**, 813–16

26. Gabriel, R. (1986). Time to scrap creatinine clearance? *Br. Med. J.* **293**, 1119–20

27. Calabrese, G., Vagelli, G. and Cristofano, C. (1982). Behaviour of arterial pressure in different stages of polycystic kidney disease. *Nephron*, **32**, 207–8

28. Mitcheson, H.D., Williams, G., Castro, J.E. (1977). Clinical aspects of polycystic disease of the kidneys. *Br. Med. J.* **1**, 1196–9

29. Reeders, S.T., Breuning, M.H., Corney, G., Jeremiah, S.J., Meera Khan, P., Davies, K.E., Hopkinson, D.A., Pearson, P.L., Weatherall, D.J. (1986). Two genetic markers closely linked to adult polycystic kidney disease on chromosome 16. *Br. Med. J.* **292**, 851–2

30. Duggan, M.L. (1963). Acute renal infarction. *J. Urol.* **90**, 669–776

31. Lessman, R.K., Johnson, S.F., Cobura, J.W., Kaufman, J.S. (1978). Renal artery embolism: Clinical features and long term follow up of 77 cases. *Ann. Intern. Med.* **89**, 477–82
32. Elkik, F., Corvol, P., Idatte, J.M., Menard, J. (1984). Renal segmental infarction: a cause of reversible malignant hypertension. *J. Hypertension* **2**, 149–56
33. Rudnick, M.R., Maxwell, M.H. (1984). Diagnosis of renovascular hypertension: limitations of renin assays. In Narins, R.G. (ed.) *Controversies in Nephrology and Hypertension*, pp 128–129. New York: Churchill Livingstone
34. Sellars, L., Shore, A.C., Wilkinson, R. (1985). Renal vein renin studies in renovascular hypertension – do they really help? *J. Hypertension* **3**, 177–81
35. Mackay, A., Boyle, P., Brown, J.J., Cumming, A.M.M., Forrest, H., Graham, A.G., Lever, A.F., Robertson, J.I.S., Semple, P.F. (1983). The decision on surgery in renal artery stenosis. *Q. J. Med.* **207**, 363–81
36. Geyskes, G.G., Puylaert, C.B.A., Oei, H.Y., Mees, E.J.D. (1983). Follow up study of 70 patients with renal artery stenosis treated by percutaneous transluminal dilatation. *Br. Med. J.* **287**, 333–6
37. Pickering, T.G., Sos, T.A., Vaughan, E.D., Case, D.B., Sealey, J.E., Harshfield, G.A., Laragh, J.H. (1984). Predictive value and changes of renal secretion in hypertensive patients with unilateral renovascular disease undergoing successful renal angioplasty. *Am. J. Med.* **76**, 398–404
38. Eyler, W.R., Clark, M.D., Garman, J.E., Rian, R.L., Meininger, D.E. (1962). Angiography of the renal areas including a comparative study of renal arterial stenosis in patients with and without hypertension. *Radiology* **78**, 879–91
39. Holley, K.E., Hunt, J.C., Brown, A.L. (1964). Renal artery stenosis – a clinical-pathological study in normotensive and hypertensive patients. *Am. J. Med.* **37**, 14–22
40. Isles, C.J. (1987). Personal communication
41. Sos, T.A., Pickering, T.G., Sniderman, K., Saddekin, S., Case, D.B., Silane, M.F., Vaughan, E.D. and Laragh, J.H. (1983). Percutaneous transluminal renal angioplasty in renovascular hypertension due to atheroma or fibromuscular dysplasia. *N. Engl. J. Med.* **309**, 274–9
42. Schreiber, M.J., Novick, A.C., Pohl, M.A. (1981). The natural history of atherosclerotic and fibrous renal artery disease. *Kidney Int.* **19**, 175
43. Hunt, J.C., Strong, C.G. (1973). Renovascular hypertension – mechanisms, natural history and treatment. *Am. J. Cardiol.* **32**, 562–74
44. Pickering, T.G., Sos, T.A., Orenstein, A., Laragh, J.H. (1986). *11th Scientific Meeting of International Society of Hypertension*, Abstract 1099
45. Sniderman, K.W., Sos, T.A. (1982). Percutaneous transluminal recanalisation and dilatation of totally occluded renal arteries. *Radiology* **142**, 607–10
46. Pickering, Tg., Sos, T.A., Laragh, J.H. (1984). Role of balloon dilatation in the treatment of renovascular hypertension. *Am. J. Med.* **77** (Suppl. 2A), 61–6
47. Shaw, A.B., Gopalka, S.K. (1982). Renal artery thrombosis caused by antihypertensive treatment. *Br. Med. J.* **285**, 1617
48. Hoefnagels, W.H.L., Thien, T. (1986). Renal artery occlusion in patients with renovascular hypertension treated with captopril. *Br. Med. J.* **292**, 24–5
49. Hricik, D.E., Browning, P.J., Kopelman, R., Goorno, W.E., Madias, N.E., Dzau, V.J. (1983). Captopril-induced functional renal insufficiency in patients with bilateral renal artery stenosis or renal artery stenosis in a solitary kidney. *N. Engl. J. Med.* **308**, 373–6

50. Watson, M.L., Bell, G.M., Muir, A.L., Buist, T.A.S., Kellett, R.J., Padfield, P.L. (1983). Captopril/diuretic combination in severe renovascular disease: a cautionary tale. *Lancet* **2**, 404–5
51. Wenting, G.J., Tan-Tjiong, H.L., Derkx, F.H.M., de Bruyn, J.H.B. Man in't Veld AJ and Schalekamp MADH. (1984). Split renal function after captopril in unilateral renal artery stenosis. *Br. Med. J.* **288**, 886–90
52. Ishikawa, K. (1978). Natural history and classification of occlusive thromboarteropathy (Takayasu's disease). *Circulation* **57**, 27–35
53. Thurm, R.H., Alexander, J.C. (1984). Captopril in the treatment of scleroderma renal crisis. *Arch. Intern. Med.* **144**, 733–5
54. Traub, Y.M., Shapiro, A.P., Rodman, G.P., Medsger, T.A., McDonald, R.H., Steen, U.D., Osial, T.A., Tolchin, S.F. (1983). Hypertension and renal failure (scleroderma renal crisis) in progressive systemic sclerosis. *Medicine* **62**, 335–52
55. Hodsman, G.P., Robertson, J.I.S. (1983). Captopril: five years on. *Br. Med. J.*, **287**, 851–2
56. Todd, P.A., Heal, R.C. (1986). Enalapril: a review of its pharmacodynamic and pharmacokinetic properties and therapeutic use in hypertension and congestive heart failure. *Drugs* **31**, 198–248
57. Case, D.B., Wallace, J.M., Keim, J.H., Weber, M.A., Sealey, J.E., Laragh, J.H. (1977). Possible role of renin in hypertension as suggested by renin-sodium profiling and inhibition of converting enzyme. *N. Engl. J. Med.* **296**, 641–6
58. Man in't Veld, A.J., Schicht, I.M., Derkx, F.H.M., de Bruyn, J.H.B., Schalekamp, M.A.D.H. (1980). Effects of angiotensin-converting enzyme inhibitor (captopril) on blood pressure. *Br. Med. J.* **280**, 288–90
59. Thurston, H., Swales, J.D. (1977). Blood-pressure response of nephrectomised hypertensive rats to converting enzyme inhibitors: evidence for persisting vascular renin activity. *Clin. Sci. Mol. Med.* **53**, 299–304
60. Leading article. (1980). Captopril: benefits and risks in severe hypertension. *Lancet* **2**, 129–30
61. Dombey, S. (1983). Optimal dosage of captopril in hypertension. *Lancet* **1**, 529
62. Isles, C.G. Hodsman, G.P., Robertson, J.I.S. (1983). Side effects of captopril. *Lancet* **1**, 355
63. McFate Smith, W., Kulaga, S.F., Moncloa, F., Pingeon, R., Walker, J.F. (1984). Overall tolerance and safety of enalapril. *J. Hypertension* **2** (Suppl. 2), 113–17
64. Hodsman, G.P., Isles, C.G., Murray, G.D., Usherwood, T.P., Webb, D.J., Robertson, J.I.S. (1983). Factors related to first dose hypotensive effect of captopril: prediction and treatment. *Br. Med. J.* **286**, 832–4
65. Webster, J., Newnham, D.M., Petrie, J.C. (1985). Initial dose of enalapril in hypertension. *Br. Med. J.* **290**, 1623–4
66. Webster, J., Newnham, D., Robb, O.J., Petrie, J.C. (1987). Antihypertensive effect of single doses of enalapril in hypertensive patients treated with bendrofluazide. *Br. J. Clin. Pharmacol.* **23**, 151–7
67. Cleland, J.G.F., Dargie, H.J., McAlpine, H., Ball, S.G., Morton, J.J., Robertson, J.I.S., Ford, I. (1985). Severe hypotension after first doses of enalapril in heart failure. *Br. Med. J.* **291**, 1309–12
68. Curtis, J.J., Luke, R.G., Whelchel, J.D., Diethelm, A.G., James, P., Dustan, H.P. (1983). Inhibition of angiotensin-converting enzyme in renal transplant recipients with hypertension. *N. Engl. J. Med.* **308**, 377–81

69. Ghione, S., Fommei, E., Palombo, C., Giaconi, S., Mantovanelli, A., Ragawzini, A., and Palla, L. (1985–86). Kidney scintigraphy after ACE inhibition in the diagnosis of renovascular hypertension. *Uraemia Invest.* **9**, 211–15

70. Silas, J.H., Klenka, Z., Solomon, S.A., Bone, J.M. (1983). Captopril induced reversible renal failure: a marker of renal artery stenosis affecting a solitary kidney. *Br. Med. J.* **286**, 1702–3

71. Enalapril in Hypertension Study Group (UK). Enalapril in essential hypertension: a comparative study with propranolol. (1984). *Br. J. Clin. Pharmacol.* **18**, 51–6

72. Webster, J., Petrie, J.C., Robb, O.J., Trafford, J., Burgess, J., Richardson, P.J., Davidson, C., Fairhurst, G., Vandenberg, M.J., Cooper, W.D., Arr, S.M., Kimber, G. (1986). Enalapril in moderate to severe hypertension: a comparison with atenolol. *Br. J. Clin. Pharmacol.* **21**, 489–95

73. Croog, S.H., Lewis, S., Testa, M.A., Brown, B., Bulpitt, C.J., Jenkins, D., Kleman, G.L., Williams, G.H. (1986). The effects of antihypertensive therapy on the quality of life. *N. Engl. J. Med.* **314**, 1657–64

74. Tillman, D.M., Malatino, L.S., Cumming, A.M.M., Hodsman, G.P., Leckie, B.J., Lever, A.F., Morton, J.J., Webb, D.J., Robertson, J.I.S. (1984). Enalapril in hypertension with renal artery stenosis: long-term follow-up and effects on renal function. *J. Hypertension* **2** (Suppl. 2), 93–100

75. Nayler, W.G., McInnes, J., Swann, J.B., Carson, V., Lowe, T.E. (1967). Effects of propranolol, a beta-adrenergic antagonist, on blood flow in the coronary and other vascular fields. *Am. Heart J.* **73**, 207–16

76. Ibsen, H., Sederberg-Olsen, P. (1973). Changes in glomerular filtration rate during long-term treatment with propranolol in patients with arterial hypertension. *Clin. Sci.* **44**, 129–34

77. Pritchard, B.N.C., Gillam, P.M.S. (1969). Treatment of hypertension with propranolol. *Br. Med. J.* **1**, 7–16

78. Warren, D.J., Swainson, C.P., Wright, N. (1974). Deterioration in renal function after beta-blockade in patients with chronic renal failure and hypertension. *Br. Med. J.* **2**, 193–4

79. Robb, O.J., Petrie, J.C., Webster, J., Harry, J. (1985). ICI 118551 does not reduce BP in hypertensive patients responsive to atenolol and propranolol. *Br. J. Clin. Pharmacol.* **19**, 541p–2p.

80. Deacon, S.P., Barnett, D. (1976). Comparison of atenolol and propranolol during insulin-induced hypoglycaemia. *Br. Med. J.* **2**, 272–3

81. Lager, I., Blomhme, G., Smith, H. (1979). Effect of cardioselective and non-selective β-blockade on the hypoglycaemic response in insulin-dependent diabetes. *Lancet* **1**, 458–62

82. Jeffers, T.A., Webster, J., Petrie, J.C., Barker, N.P. (1977). Atenolol once-daily in hypertension. *Br. J. Clin. Pharmacol.* **4**, 523–7

83. Webster, J., Petrie, J.C., Robb, O.J., Jamieson, M., Verschueren, J. (1985). A comparison of single doses of bucindolol and oxprenolol in hypertensive patients. *Br. J. Clin. Pharmacol.* **20**, 393–400

84. Bannan, L.T. and Beevers, D.G. (1981). Emergency treatment of high blood pressure with oral atenolol. *Br. Med. J.* **282**, 1757–8

85. Pritchard, B.N.C. Beta-adrenoceptor blocking agents. In Abshagen, U. (Ed.) *Clinical Pharmacology of Antianginal Drugs.* Handbook of Experimental Pharmacology, vol. 76, pp. 385–485. (Berlin: Springer)

37

86. Lowenthal, D.T. (1977). Pharmacokinetics of propranolol, quinidine, pro-cainamide and lidocaine in chronic renal disease. *Am. J. Med.* **62**, 532–8
87. Johnsson, G., Regardh, C-G. (1976). Clinical pharmacokinetics of β-adreno-ceptor blocking drugs. *Clin. Pharmacokinet.* **1**, 233–63
88. Sorkin, E.M., Clissold, S.P., Brogden, R.N. (1985). Nifedipine: a review of its pharmacodynamic and pharmacokinetic properties and therapeutic efficacy in ischaemic heart disease, hypertension and related cardiovascular disorders. *Drugs* **30**, 182–274
89. Lee, S.M., Williams, R., Warnock, D., Emmett, M., Wolbach, R.A. (1986). The effects of nicardipine in hypertensive subjects with impaired renal function. *Br. J. Clin. Pharmacol.* **22**, 297s–306s
90. Diamond, J.R., Cheung, J.Y., Fang, L.S.T. (1984). Nifedipine-induced renal dysfunction. *Am. J. Med.* **77**, 905–9
91. Mroczek, W.J., Leibel, B.A., Davidov, M., Finnerty, F.A. (1971). The import-ance of the rapid administration of diazoxide in accelerated hypertension. *N. Engl. J. Med.* **285**, 803–6
92. Ledingham, J.G.G., Rajagopalan, B. (1979). Cerebral complications in the treatment of accelerated hypertension. *Q. Med. J.* **48**, 25–41
93. Thien, T.A., Huysmans, F.T.M., Gerlag, P.G.G., Koene, R.A.P., Wijdeveld, P.G.A.B. (1979). Diazoxide infusion in severe hypertension and hypertensive crisis. *Clin. Pharmacol. Ther.* **25**, 795–9
94. O'Malley, K., Velasco, M., Pruitt, A., McNay, J.L. (1975). Decreased plasma protein binding of diazoxide in uraemia. *Clin. Pharmacol. Ther.* **18**, 53–8
95. Koch-Weser, J. (1976). Diazoxide. *N. Engl. J. Med.* **294**, 1271–4
96. Bennett, W.H., McDonald, W.J., Kuehnel, E., Hartnett, M.H., Porter, G.A. (1977). Do diuretics have antihypertensive properties independent of natriuresis? *Clin. Pharmacol. Ther.* **22**, 499–504
97. Tobian, L. (1967). Why do thiazide diuretics lower blood pressure in essential hypertension? *Annu. Rev. Pharmacol.* **7**, 399–408
98. Webster, J. (1985). Interactions of NSAIDs with diuretics and β-blockers. Mechanisms and clinical implications. *Drugs* **30**, 32–41
99. Jones, B. and Nanra, R.S. (1979). Double-blind trial of antihypertensive effects of chlorothiazide in severe renal failure. *Lancet* **2**, 1258–60
100. Ram, C.V.S., Garrett, B.N., Kaplan, W.M. (1981). Moderate sodium restriction and various diuretics in the treatment of hypertension: effect of potassium wastage and blood pressure control. *Arch. Intern. Med.* **141**, 1015–19
101. Weiner, I.M., Mudge, G.H. (1985). Diuretics and other agents employed in the mobilisation of edema fluid. In Gilman, A.G., Goodman, L.S., Rall, T.W., Murad, F. (Eds.) The Pharmacological Basis of Therapeutics, 7th Edn., pp. 887–907. New York: Macmillan
102. Sorkin, E.M., Brogden, R.N., Romankiewicz, J.A. (1984). Intravenous glyceryl trinitrate (Nitroglycerin). A review of its pharmacological properties and thera-peutic efficacy. *Drugs* **27**, 45–80
103. Cameron, H.A., Ramsay, L.E. (1984). The lupus syndrome induced by hydrala-zine: a common complication with lower dose treatment. *Br. Med. J.* **289**, 410–12
104. McAreavey, D., Ramsay, L.E., Latham, L., McLaren, A.D., Lorimer, A.R., Reid, J.L., Robertson, J.I.S., Robertson, M.P., Weir, R.J. (1984). "Third drug" trial: comparative study of antihypertensive agents added to treatment when

blood pressure remains uncontrolled by a beta blocker plus thiazide diuretic. *Br. Med. J.* **288**, 106–10

105. Talseth, T. (1976). Studies on hydralazine. II Elimination rate and steady-state concentration in patients with impaired renal function. *Eur. J. Clin. Pharmacol.* **10**, 311–17

106. Webster, J., Jeffers, T.A., Galloway, D.B., Petrie, J.C., Barker, N.P. (1977). Atenolol, methyldopa and chlorthalidone in moderate hypertension. *Br. Med. J.* **1**, 76–7

107. Myhre, E., Rugstad, H.E., Hansen, T. (1982). Clinical pharmacokinetics of methyldopa. *Clin. Pharmacokinet.* **7**, 221–33

108. Dargie, H.J., Dollery, C.T., Daniel, J. (1977). Minoxidil in resistant hypertension. *Lancet* **2**, 515–18

109. Devine, B.L., Fife, R., Trust, P.M. (1977). Minoxidil for severe hypertension after failure of other hypotensive drugs. *Br. Med. J.* **2**, 667–9

110. Lowenthal, D.T., Affrime, M.B. (1980). Pharmacology and pharmacokinetics of minoxidil. *J. Cardiovasc. Pharmacol.* **2** (Suppl. 2), S93–S106

111. Page, I.H., Corcoran, A.C., Dunstan, H.P., Koppanyi, T. (1955). Cardiovascular action of sodium nitroprusside in animals and hypertensive patients. *Circulation* **11**, 188–98

112. Russell, G.I., Bing, R.F., Swales, J.D. (1978). Sodium nitroprusside and renovascular hypertension. *Br. Med. J.* **2**, 14

113. Stanaszek, W.F., Kellerman, D., Brogden, R.N. and Romankiewicz, J.A. (1983). Prazosin update. A review of its pharmacological properties and therapeutic use in hypertension and congestive heart failure. *Drugs* **25**, 339–84

114. Collier, J.C., Lorge, R.E., Robinson, B.F. (1978). Comparison of effects of tolmesoxide (RX 71107) diazoxide, hydralazine, prazosin, glyceryl trinitrate and sodium nitroprusside on forearm arteries and dorsal hand veins of man. *Br. J. Clin. Pharmacol.* **5**, 35–44

115. Graham, R.M., Thornell, J.R., Gain, J.M., Bagnoli, C., Oates, H.F., Stokes, G.S. (1976). Prazosin: The first dose phenomenon. *Br. Med. J.* **2**, 1293

116. Velasco, M., Silva, H., Morillo, J., Pellieir, R., Urbina-Quintana, A., Hernandez-Pieretti, O. (1981). Effect of prazosin on blood lipids and on thyroid function in hypertensive patients. *J. Cardiovasc. Pharmacol.* **3**, (Suppl. 3), 193–7

117. Stokes, G.S., Monaghan, J.C., Frost, G.W., MacCarthy, E.P. (1979). Responsiveness to prazosin in renal failure. *Clin. Sci.* **57**, 383s–5s

118. Chin, D.K.F., Ho, A.K.C., Tse, C.Y. (1986). Neuropsychiatric complications related to use of prazosin in patients with renal failure. *Br. Med. J.* **293**, 1347

119. Lee, C.C., Marburg, T.C. (1984). Drug therapy in patients undergoing haemodialysis. Clinical pharmacokinetic considerations. *Clin. Pharmacokinet.* **9**, 42–66

120. Kuntzinger, H., Pouthier, D., Belluci, A. (1986). Treatment of hypertension with lisinopril in end-stage renal failure. *11th Scientific Meeting of the International Society of Hypertension*, Abstract No 532.

2
MALIGNANT HYPERTENSION

C. G. ISLES

INTRODUCTION

Clinicians who manage patients with malignant hypertension (MHT) have witnessed some remarkable changes in recent years. The incidence of the disease appears to have fallen, at least in the U.K. and other Western countries[1]. Reduction of blood pressure within minutes by parenteral therapy is no longer recommended as a routine procedure, and it is now recognized that initial management is best achieved by one or two drugs given orally in most cases[2]. Moreover, survival has improved as a result of more effective antihypertensive drug therapy and the increasing availability of renal dialysis and transplantation[3-6].

Despite these encouraging trends, a number of difficult areas persist. MHT continues to be a major problem in developing countries and is likely to remain so for some time[7]. Also of concern is the fact that as the disease becomes less common in the West, too few doctors see enough of its complications, especially hypertensive encephalopathy, to gain expertise in its management[2]. Moreover, despite the overall improvement in survival rate, the prognosis for patients with significant impairment of renal function remains poor[3-6].

This chapter deals with the pathogenesis, clinical features and prognosis of MHT, and in particular with recent developments. It also includes a survey of 139 patients with MHT who were seen in Glasgow between 1968 and 1983.

DIAGNOSTIC CRITERIA

The new WHO criteria are probably the most useful, namely that patients diagnosed as having malignant hypertension should have severe hypertension with bilateral retinal haemorrhages and exudates[8]. Diastolic blood pressure is usually greater than 130 mmHg, but there is no absolute level above which MHT always develops and below which it never occurs. Lower blood pressures are said to be characteristic of patients with eclampsia and acute glomerulo-nephritis[9], although both are uncommon in the U.K. today, and of patients with renal failure[10]. Conversely, patients are frequently seen with blood pressures greater than 130 mmHg who do not have MHT[11]. Other features of the disease, such as microangiopathic haemolytic anaemia (MAHA) or renal failure, need not always be present.

A heated debate has been conducted over the years concerning the severity of the fundal changes necessary to establish the diagnosis of MHT. At one extreme, the view has been expressed[9] that 'one large exudate convicts'. Others have argued that hypertension should not be classified as malignant unless papilloedema is present[12,13], preferring to use the term 'accelerated' hypertension to describe patients with retinal haemorrhages and exudates alone[14]. It is the view of the Glasgow MRC unit that papilloedema need not be present in MHT, and in support of this I would cite the following evidence. First, fibrinoid arteriolar necrosis has been detected in hypertensive patients with haemorrhages and exudates alone[15]. Second, soft exudates and papilloedema share a similar pathogenesis[16]. Third, papilloedema is not constantly present even when MHT causes acute oliguric renal failure, one of the most malignant of all presentations of hyper-tension[17]. Fourth, it has been shown recently that papilloedema is of no additional prognostic importance in patients treated for hypertension who already have bilateral haemorrhages and exudates[18,19].

This long-standing argument will, it is hoped, now be settled. Agree-ment on the diagnosis of MHT is important for epidemiological purposes and, for the reasons outlined above, the WHO criteria have been adopted in Glasgow. In practice, however, one would never wait for the full syndrome to occur, and the development of fresh haemorrhages or soft exudates in a hypertensive patient, either *de novo* or when blood pressure is poorly controlled, signifies an urgent need for effective treatment.

PATHOLOGY

Although fibrinoid arteriolar necrosis is usually regarded as the histological hallmark of the acute stage of the disease, this lesion is not pathognomonic for MHT nor is it necessarily the most significant finding[11,20]. Subintimal cellular proliferation of the interlobular arteries of the kidney is seen more commonly and could be important in its own right, because intimal thickening in these small arteries may be so great as to occlude their lumina (Figure 2.1). It is likely that this type of damage to vessels plays a major part in causing the chronic renal ischaemia, and thus the chronic renal failure, that so often accompanies MHT[11].

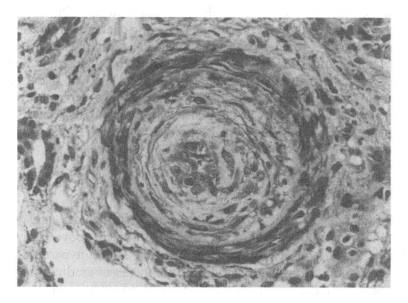

FIGURE 2.1 Renal biopsy in MHT showing marked subintimal cellular proliferation of an interlobular artery. The vessel lumen appears to have been completely occluded by the thickened intima.

PATHOGENESIS

The cycle of events leading to these pathological changes is still not fully understood. Most would accept that increased arterial pressure is the primary event and that the rate of rise of pressure is more important than the actual level achieved, but opinion is divided on whether there are other factors capable of determining which patients will enter the malignant phase. Some have argued that increased arterial pressure is the only factor[21], while others believe that immunological changes[22], intravascular coagulation[23,24], cigarette-smoking[25,26], the oral contraceptive pill[27] and vasoactive agents[28,29] may play important though subsidiary roles.

Whichever of these hypotheses is true, and it should be emphasized that they are not mutually exclusive, the appearance of alternating bands of constriction and dilatation in arterioles (the so called 'sausage-string' effect) probably heralds the onset of MHT[11]. It is likely that the dilated segments represent focal failure of the vessel wall to resist a rapid rise in intraluminal pressure, and it has been shown that these areas are abnormally permeable to plasma proteins[30]. Disruption of the vessel wall may then trigger the following changes: insudation of plasma, leading to deposition of fibrin, i.e. fibrinoid necrosis[30]; platelet aggregation, causing release of growth factors that could well cause the subintimal cellular proliferation[31]; and activation of the coagulation system[23]. The last may promote further deposition of fibrin, not only in the vessel wall but also within the microcirculation, thereby causing microangiopathic haemolytic anaemia[32].

EPIDEMIOLOGY

MHT can occur in patients of any age but rarely does so in those older than seventy years. For the reasons outlined above, this is probably because MHT is most likely when severe hypertension develops rapidly. If, instead, blood pressure increases gradually over many years to reach very high levels at an advanced age, the vasculature may have time to adapt and so avoid the disruption that leads to subintimal cellular proliferation and fibrinoid necrosis[33].

Most[3,6,7,12,13] but not all[4,5] studies show a preponderance of males

44

among sufferers. Also, the disease seems commoner in Blacks than Whites[34]. Indeed, while many authors now consider MHT to be rare among Whites[1] it remains a common problem in developing countries; in a recent report from Johannesburg, no fewer than 2% of all admissions to the medical wards of the 'Non-European' hospital were because of MHT[7].

UNDERLYING CAUSES

It is well recognized that patients with MHT are more likely to have an underlying cause for their high blood pressure than are patients with non-malignant hypertension. Renal and renovascular diseases are those most commonly identified[3-6,35], although any cause of raised blood pressure can lead to the malignant phase if the hypertension is severe enough and if the blood pressure has risen so rapidly as to exceed the autoregulatory capacity of the retinal circulation. Even patients with Conn's syndrome, a condition generally assocated with mild-to-moderate hypertension, may occasionally develop the malignant phase[36,37].

The proportion of patients with MHT who are found to have an

Table 2.1   Underlying causes of malignant hypertension

	Glasgow	Melbourne	Leicester	Johannes-burg Blacks	Vanderbilt Whites
Period of study	1968–83	1979–85	1974–83	1979–80	1964–77
Number of patients	139	83	100	62	76
Essential	60	20	68	82	?
Renal	18	46	19	5	?
Renovascular	14	13	6	3	32
Other	9	21	7	10	?

Table shows percentage of patients with possible underlying causes for MHT in different centres. The data for the Vanderbilt series is incomplete except for the group with renovascular disease. Detailed references are given in the text underlying cause for their hypertension varies markedly in different series (Table 2.1). This is likely to reflect real differences in the prevalence of some diseases (e.g. IgA nephropathy and analgesic nephropathy, which are particularly common in Australia) as well as the enthusiasm of the diagnostic search and the specific interests of individual units. The high prevalence of malignant essential hypertension among Johannesburg Blacks[7] has been confirmed by autopsy studies[38] suggesting that racial factors may also be important.

When investigating hypertensives for an underlying cause, it should be borne in mind that occasional patients only can be cured of their hypertension by specific intervention whereas most patients with renal impairment have irreversible disease and a particularly high risk of premature vascular death[39]. This is even more likely to be true of malignant hypertension than of non-malignant hypertension, since renal causes are found more commonly in the former. Therefore, at least as much emphasis should be placed on control of blood pressure and reduction of associated vascular risks (particularly cigarette-smoking) as on the pursuit pathology in such patients.

Other factors which may influence the development of MHT

Cigarette-smoking

The relation between cigarette-smoking and hypertension is intriguing. Epidemiological studies show an inverse relation between smoking and blood pressure[40] and yet the act of smoking causes a transient rise in pressure[41]. The increased mortality rate among smokers with hypertension is also well known[42]. The first suggestion that smoking may predispose to MHT in patients who are already hypertensive came in 1979, when workers in Glasgow and Birmingham reported that MHT occurred five times more often in hypertensives who smoked than in hypertensives who did not smoke[25,26]. Similar findings have subsequently been reported from other centres[43,44].

An interesting exception to this trend is the study from Johannesburg[7], in which cigarette-smoking was not a feature of the behaviour of urban Blacks with MHT, in whom, as described previously, the disease appears to be particularly common. Clearly, then, smoking is not the cause of MHT. The possibility remains that smoking could act as a trigger in susceptible patients, and that it exerts its effect by promoting intravascular coagulation[45]. Alternatively, smoking may be a marker for some other variable that is itself a cause of MHT. Hypertensives with negative attitudes to health may be more likely to default from clinic attendance and less likely to comply with therapy, and may thus be predisposed to develop the malignant phase. Such patients may also be more likely to smoke. This area deserves further study.

The oral contraceptive pill

The oral contraceptive pill causes a small rise in blood pressure in most women and a large rise in blood pressure in a few. A number of case reports have documented an association between oral contraceptives and MHT[27,46–51] and in a series from Glasgow no fewer than 32% of women with MHT who were of child-bearing age were taking the pill at the time of diagnosis[52]. There are, however, epidemiological difficulties with this type of analysis, because the lack of adequate controls precludes a reliable estimate of the number of pill users in the general population. Nevertheless, a causal association seems likely when patients who were previously known to be normotensive develop MHT within a few weeks or months of starting to take oral contraceptives, even if, as is usually the case, their blood pressure does not fall to normal when the pill is stopped. Although it is generally agreed that the risk of MHT is less with low-oestrogen pills, we have seen a patient who was previously normotensive and who presented with MHT within eight weeks of starting to take a pill containing only $20\,\mu g$ ethinyloestradiol. No other cause for her hypertension was found[52].

MHT may develop as a consequence of the known pressor effects of oestrogens or progestagens or as a result of some other property of the pill. It is known that oral contraceptives activate the coagulation system[53] and that *in situ* thrombosis causes other cardiovascular complications of the pill. As already discussed, abnormalities of blood coagulation are well recognized in MHT that are not associated with oral contraceptives. It is possible, therefore, that *in situ* thrombosis involving either the main[54] or the intrarenal [55] arteries could contribute to the pathogenesis of MHT in pill users.

CLINICAL FEATURES

The wide variety of clinical features that may occur in MHT are well described in earlier reviews[12,13] and the frequency with which some of these occurred in the Glasgow series is summarized in Table 3.2.

In stark contrast to patients with non-malignant hypertension, which is essentially a symptomless condition, patients with MHT nearly always present with symptoms. Recent onset of headache and visual upset are the commonest complaints (Table 2.2)[12,13]. Although the headache of MHT is said characteristically to be worse in the mornings[14,56], there was no diurnal variation in our patients. Visual symptoms were generally related in degree to the severity of the

Table 2.2 Clinical features of malignant hypertension in Glasgow

	%
Headache	63
Visual upset	59
Mild renal impairment (serum creatinine 115–300 μmol/l)	46
Moderate and severe renal impairment (serum creatinine > 300 μmol/l)	33
Cardiac failure	30
LVH by voltage criteria	86
Neurological complications	17
Gastrointestinal symptoms	49
MAHA	28
Secondary hyperaldosteronism	76

The prevalence of headache, visual upset and gastrointestinal symptoms was estimated by questionnaire in 59 consecutive patients between 1979 and 1981. The value for MAHA is derived from 107 patients having blood films within a week of presentation, whereas the estimate for secondary hyperaldosteronism was based on 37 previously untreated patients in whom plasma active renin concentration was measured. All other values in this table are based on all 139 patients in the Glasgow series changes in the retinal and optic nerves. In addition, one patient experienced sudden loss of vision due to an associated central retinal vein thrombosis, and two presented with visual field defects due to small strokes. Visual deterioration after treatment had begun was recorded in only one patient, a 19-year-old girl who developed cortical blindness, which was transient, when her blood pressure fell precipitously with intravenous diazoxide.

Renal failure is the most serious manifestation of MHT, and moderate-to-severe renal impairment was present in 33% of the patients in Glasgow (Table 2.2). Despite investigation, it was often difficult to be certain whether hypertension preceded the renal failure or whether an underlying renal disorder caused the hypertension. Exclusion of renovascular disease is important under these circumstances, since surgical intervention in selected cases may improve both blood-pressure control and renal function[57]. Otherwise, and in the majority of cases, the distinction between primary hypertension and primary renal disease may yield useful prognostic information (see later) but does not lead to a change in management.

The heart is commonly involved in MHT, and breathlessness due to cardiac failure is a frequent clinical manifestation (Table 2.2). By contrast, ischaemic chest pain occurs rarely[13]. Left ventricular hypertrophy may be prominent[58] but is not a universal finding[59]. When left ventricular hypertrophy is absent, it is likely that MHT was of sudden onset and not preceded by a long period of non-malignant hypertension in that patient.

A number of neurological complications may occur[60,61]. The most serious of these is hypertensive encephalopathy, whose clinical hallmark is altered consciousness, ranging from agitation to coma. Other features of hypertensive encephalopathy include headache, nausea and vomiting, seizures and changing focal neurological signs. Fundal examination will usually show retinal haemorrhages, exudates or papilloedema, but this depends to some extent on the rate of rise of blood pressure. There will, however, always be marked arteriolar spasm. There may be difficulty in distinguishing hypertensive encephalopathy from cerebral haemorrhage, since severe hypertension and ischaemic retinopathy may be present in both conditions. As a general rule, patients with major lateralizing signs are more likely to have cerebral haemorrhage[60]. The distinction is important because the rate at which blood pressure should be reduced depends on the specific clinical diagnosis.

Gastrointestinal symptoms including anorexia, nausea, vomiting, abdominal pain and weight loss occurred in 49% of the Glasgow patients. The association of MHT and weight loss has been noted before and is not explained entirely by the degree of renal impairment[13]; in one of our patients it was the major feature at presentation. Abdominal pain due to acute pancreatitis[62] and small bowel infarction[63] have also been recorded.

Other well-recognized features of MHT include MAHA and secondary hyperaldosteronism. MAHA is thought to arise when red cells are fragmented upon fibrin strands that have been laid down within the microcirculation[32]. The diagnosis is based on the presence of fragmented red cells on the blood film and, when fully developed, MAHA is associated with low haemoglobin, low platelet and reticulocyte counts. In the Glasgow series, 107/139 patients had blood films during the first week of their illness and of these 28% showed red-cell fragmentation. In no instance was there clinical evidence of an abnormal bleeding tendency. Moreover, in cases where conventional coagulation screens were performed, they were always normal.

Secondary hyperaldosteronism occurs more frequently than MAHA in MHT, but again this is not a universal finding. Hypokalaemia will usually be present and is a useful clue to the diagnosis. Presumably, the renin system is activated by renal ischaemia or by sodium depletion. In the Glasgow series, elevated plasma active renin concentration was found in 76% of previously untreated patients in whom it was measured. Increased renin was of no value in differentiating the cause of the hypertension in these patients, nor was it of any prognostic significance, since there was no tendency for patients with higher renin concentrations to have higher mortality.

DIFFERENTIAL DIAGNOSIS OF HYPERTENSIVE RETINOPATHY

Accurate diagnosis depends upon thorough examination of the fundus. If an adequate view cannot be obtained in a darkened room, tropicamide drops 0.5% are recommended for their quick onset and short duration of action. Tropicamide is contraindicated in narrow-angle glaucoma but is safe in the majority of glaucomas that are open-angle. If tropicamide is not available, cyclopentolate 1%, which has a slightly slower onset and longer duration of action, may be substituted. Pilocarpine 2% can be used to reduce the period of mydriasis after the examination is complete. If one is available, a fundus photograph will further aid evaluation of the retinal appearances, but fluorescien angiography is rarely necessary.

In its most florid form, the retinae of patients with MHT display a profusion of hard and soft exudates with flame-shaped haemorrhages, macular stars and papilloedema (Figure 2.2(a)). The pathogenesis of this form of hypertensive retinopathy has been reviewed recently[64]. It is important to appreciate that these changes are characteristic but not pathognomonic of MHT, and that similar appearances may be seen in patients with diabetes mellitus, retinal vascular occlusion, raised intracranial pressure, gastrointestinal haemorrhage and a number of haematological disorders including anaemia, poly-cythaemia, leukaemia and Waldenstrom's macroglobulinaemia, all of which may produce an ischaemic retinopathy.

When dot-and-blot haemorrhages and new vessels are seen (Figure 2.2(b)) the diagnosis of diabetic retinopathy is rarely in doubt, but occasionally an ischaemic retinopathy indistinguishable from that of MHT can occur. Central retinal vein occlusion is characterized by sudden loss of vision and an engorged retina in which haemorrhage is a prominent feature (Figure 2.2(c)), whereas in branch vein occlusion all the damage is seen in the area of the affected vein (Figure 2.2(d)). It is important to differentiate vein occlusions correctly, not least because they are associated with a better prognosis[65]. Raised intra-cranial pressure may cause diagnostic difficulty and an appearance of the fundus similar to that in MHT, although venous distension is greater (Figure 2.2(e)). Gastrointestinal blood loss is another condition in which a haemorrhagic and/or exudative retinopathy of varying severity may develop that may be indistinguishable from that in MHT. Pears and Pickering[66] described seven cases, concluding that anaemia *per se* could not always be held responsible, and that the retinal changes sometimes occurred as a result of a profound though transient reduction in blood pressure. In anaemia alone, a purely haemorrhagic retinopathy is more commonly seen (Figure 2.2(f)). The fundoscopic appearances due to the other haematological disorders that can cause ischaemic retinopathy are described elsewhere[67].

The occurrence of such similar retinal changes in these apparently unrelated conditions suggests a common pathogenesis that Pears and Pickering have postulated may be focal hypoxia[66]. Thus, it may be useful to consider the retina as having a limited range of responses to a variety of different insults. In the same way that proteinuria may be the end-result of renal damage from drugs, toxins, immunological and multisystem disease, so may haemorrhages and exudates be the ultimate expression of hypertension, diabetes and other disorders that affect the retinal circulation. If this is correct, then this model may also explain the tendency for ischaemic retinopathy to develop at lower blood pressures when another disorder capable of causing ischaemic retinal damage is present. The increased incidence of exudates in diabetic patients who are hypertensive, may be an example[68], and the well-recognized tendency for ischaemic retinopathy to develop at lower pressures in renal patients[10] may be another, reflecting the combined insults of hypertension and anaemia.

INITIAL MANAGEMENT OF MALIGNANT HYPERTENSION

The ideal rate of reduction of blood pressure in patients with MHT must represent a balance between the risks of inadequate reduction and too-rapid reduction of blood pressure. Central to this is the

---

FIGURE 2.2 (a) Malignant hypertension: in this particularly florid example, hard and soft exudates, flame shaped haemorrhages, macular star and papilloedema are seen. (b) Diabetic retinopathy: dot and blot haemorrhages and hard exudates are typical, but occasionally an ischaemic retinopathy indistinguishable from that of MHT may occur. (c) Central retinal vein occlusion: an engorged retina, with haemorrhage a prominent feature, is typical. (d) Branch vein occlusion: haemorrhages and exudates are limited to the area of the affected vein. (e) Raised intracranial pressure: fundus appearance may be similar to that of MHT except that venous distension is greater. (f) Anaemia: haemorrhage is the main feature of this form of retinopathy, in this case due to pernicious anaemia

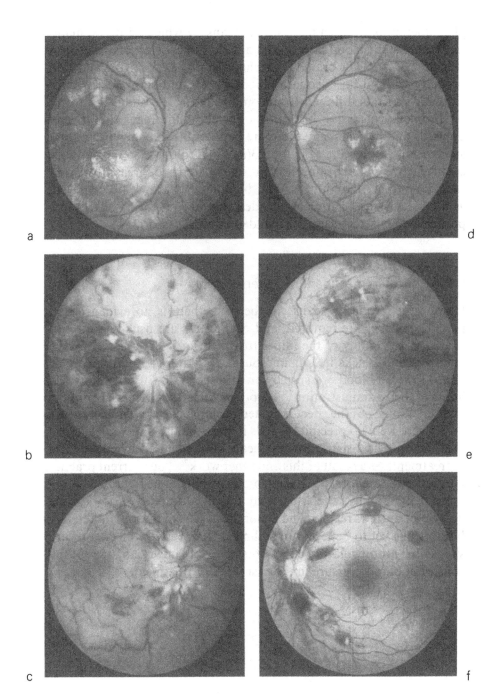

phenomenon of autoregulation, the means by which an organ maintains a constant blood flow across a wide range of arterial pressures (Figure 2.3(a))[69]. The brain in particular has little capacity to function properly without an adequate blood supply, and shows clear autoregulation of blood flow[70]. In uncomplicated MHT and other forms of chronic hypertension, the range of cerebral autoregulation is reset upwards and patients may therefore be less able to compensate for a sudden fall in pressure (Figure 2.3(b)). Neurological complications, particularly cerebral infarction in the watershed areas (so-called boundary zone infarction)[71,72] and blindness[73,74] are well recognized; as a result, it has been recommended that abrupt forms of therapy, particularly injected drugs, be avoided in most cases.

Uncomplicated malignant hypertension

Despite their widespread use in the past, there is no evidence that parenteral drugs are required, and oral agents are usually quite satisfactory. In a study of the initial treatment of uncomplicated MHT among urban Blacks in Johannesburg, both atenolol and nifedipine retard lowered blood pressure by an average of 20–30% within a few hours of their administration[75]. Blood pressure decreased more rapidly after nifedipine but the effect persisted for longer after atenolol (Figure 2.4). There were no precipitous falls in pressure; no patient developed focal neurological signs; nor was heart failure caused by either form of treatment. As a result of this and other work[76,77] our current practice is to prescribe atenolol 50–100 mg orally or nifedipine retard 20–40 mg twice daily initially, and usually to add in a diuretic on the second day. Some authors recommend a diuretic as part of the initial therapy[2], but this has yet to be tested in a clinical trial. In light of the upward shift in the autoregulatory curve, it is probably unwise to attempt full control of blood pressure in the first week of treatment.

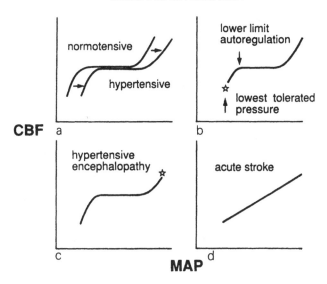

CBF

FIGURE 2.3 Relation between cerebral blood flow (CBF) and mean arterial pressure (MAP). In normotensive man, CBF is maintained at 50 ml per 100 g/min across a wide range of arterial pressure from 65 to 140 mmHg. In hypertension, the curve is reset upwards (*a*). The lower limit of autoregulation is the point at which CBF begins to fall and the lowest tolerated pressure the point at which symptoms of cerebral ischaemia are likely to develop. The brain can compensate to some extent for the loss of flow by extracting more oxygen from the blood. Nevertheless it follows that symptoms of cerebral ischaemia are more likely to occur in hypertensive patients whose blood pressures are reduced too quickly (*b*). In hypertensive encephalopathy the rate of rise of blood pressure is thought to have been so rapid as to have exceeded the upper limit of autoregulation, causing hyperperfusion, cerebral oedema and, if untreated, death (*c*). Cerebral autoregulation is lost in the area of an acute stroke so that CBF to the ischaemic area becomes pressure-dependent (*d*).

Malignant hypertension with renal failure

It used to be recommended that blood pressure be lowered cautiously in patients with MHT and renal failure[78], since acute loss of renal function resulting from rapid lowering of blood pressure was commonly fatal before dialysis became generally available. Opinion has changed recently and recommendations for patients with renal failure

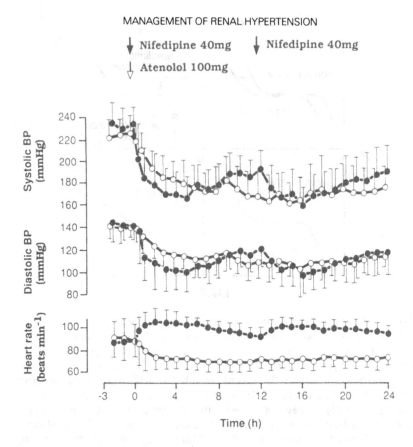

FIGURE 2.4   Blood pressure (means ± S.D.) and heart rate after nifedipine retard (solid circles) and atenolol (open circles) in study of initial
treatment of MHT in Blacks[75]. The fall in systolic and diastolic pressure,
and the change in heart rate, were significant ($p < 0.01$) at all times after
1 h in both treatment groups

are now the same as for uncomplicated MHT. The rationale is that
renal failure will worsen unless the vessel changes can be made to heal,
and that this can only be done by reducing the blood pressure[79]. As
far as individual drugs are concerned, parenteral hydralazine not only
appears to be more effective in renal failure than when renal function
is normal, but is also associated with a relative sparing of renal blood
flow, so that this drug is commonly used in patients with renal failure
who are unable to take oral medication[14]. It should also be borne in

mind that some β-receptor antagonists, e.g. atenolol, accumulate in renal failure, and that thiazide diuretics become less effective when serum creatinine concentration is greater than 200 μmol/l. It is not unusual to need large doses, 250–1000 mg daily, of frusemide in order to control blood pressure and/or fluid retention in patients with renal failure.

Hypertensive heart failure

Hypertensive heart failure differs from other forms of cardiac failure in that drug treatment not only relieves symptoms but also removes the underlying cause, namely increased afterload. It generally responds to conventional treatment with diuretics and vasodilators such as oral nifedipine or hydralazine. Reflex tachycardia is rarely a problem, since the sympathetic nervous system is already maximally stimulated. Although ACE inhibitors have also been recommended and should theoretically be of value[80,81], a precipitous fall in blood pressure is quite likely to occur after the first dose when plasma renin concentration is high (as in MHT or in patients already taking large doses of diuretics) and these drugs are probably best avoided in the acute phase. When life-threatening and accompanied by pulmonary oedema, hypertensive heart failure should be treated with intravenous morphine, intravenous diuretics and oxygen, together with intravenous nitroprusside or nitroglycerine in order to achieve rapid and controlled reduction of blood pressure (Table 2.3)[82].

Hypertensive encephalopathy

In hypertensive encephalopathy the rate of rise of blood pressure is thought to have exceeded the upper limit of autoregulation, causing hyperperfusion, cerebral oedema and, if untreated, cerebral haemorrhage and death (Figure 2.3(c))[83]. Fortunately, it is extremely uncommon, but as a consequence of this, few doctors in Europe, America and Australia see sufficient numbers of patients with hypertensive encephalopathy to gain much experience in its management.

The drug of choice is one with rapid onset of action, causing

Table 2.3 Antihypertensive drugs for parenteral administration

Drug	Preferred route and dose range	Onset and duration of action	Comments
Nitroprusside	0.5–8 μg kg^{-1} min^{-1} by i.v. infusion	onset instantaneous, duration 2–3 min after infusion stopped	requires careful monitoring (see text); particularly useful in heart failure
Hydralazine	20 mg in 20 ml at 1 mg/min by i.v. bolus	onset 10–20 min, duration 4–6 h	avoid in IHD; reflex tachycardia can be prevented by addition of 1–10 mg propranolol i.v.; particularly useful in renal failure; can also be given i.m.
Labetalol	2 mg/min to total of 2 mg/kg by i.v. infusion	onset 5–10 min; duration 1–8 h after infusion stopped	avoid in cardiac failure, asthma, second or third degree heart block; β-blocking effects predominate; reflex tachycardia does not occur; can also be given by incremental infusion[85]
Diazoxide	50–100 mg given rapidly by i.v. bolus every 10–15 min	onset within 5 min; duration up to 18 h	avoid in IHD; reflex tachycardia as per hydralazine; may cause hyperglycaemia; precipitous falls in pressure recorded with 300 mg i.v. bolus dose
Nitroglycerin	0.5–8 μg kg^{-1} min^{-1} by i.v. infusion	onset within minutes; duration 2–3 min after infusion stopped	particularly useful in acute MI or heart failure; administer by syringe pump (drug absorbed by soft plastic containers)
Phentolamine	5 mg every 5 min to total of 20 mg by i.v. bolus, then 1 mg/min by i.v. infusion	onset instantaneous; duration 5–10 min after bolus dose or infusion stopped	should only be used when phaeochromocytoma present or suspected side-effects include reflex tachycardia and cardiac arrythmias
Trimethaphan	1–15 mg/min by i.v. infusion	onset 5–10 min; duration 5–10 min after infusion stopped	still used occasionally for dissecting aneurysms, and in combination with nitroprusside (see text); head-up tilt augments antihypertensive effect; side-effects of ganglion blockade, especially urinary retention and paralytic ileus, make it inappropriate to use this drug for more than 48 h may also cause deterioration of renal function

58

predictable fall in blood pressure, with short duration of therapeutic effect and preservation of cerebral blood flow; the drug that fulfils most of these criteria is nitroprusside[84]. Although it is widely recommended, particular care has to be taken with this drug, which is inactivated by light and must be given by constant intravenous infusion. The hypotensive effect of nitroprusside is so short-lived that if the infusion is interrupted for any reason, blood pressure will very quickly return to baseline levels. Moreover, nitroprusside has a toxic metabolite, thiocyanate, that is excreted by the kidneys. This limits use of the drug in patients with renal failure in whom thiocyanate psychosis, a syndrome that resembles hypertensive encephalopathy, may develop[82]. During prolonged infusion, blood thiocyanate should be measured daily after 48 hours, and the infusion should be stopped if the level exceeds $12 \, mg\%$[14]. For these reasons, nitroprusside should probably only be given when intensive care facilities are available. The usual starting dose is $0.5 \, \mu g \, kg^{-1} \, min^{-1}$, e.g. 100 mg nitroprusside in 250 ml saline at 5–10 ml/h. In patients who require infusion rates of more than 30 ml/h, 50 mg nitroprusside may be combined with 250 mg trimethaphan in 250 ml saline to give the same degree of efficacy but with fewer side-effects.

Experience in Glasgow with labetalol given by intravenous infusion suggests that this might be a useful alternative treatment for hypertensive encephalopathy[85]. Intravenous hydralazine and diazoxide have also been recommended (Table 2.3)[82]. Nifedipine 10 mg given sublingually every 4–6 hours has the attraction of simplicity and may be a safe alternative to parenteral therapy[77]. Drugs such as reserpine, clonidine and methyldopa are not recommended, because they cause drowsiness and thereby make the patients' conscious level more difficult to assess. Intravenous diazepam is indicated for patients with seizures, although reduction of blood pressure alone may also be effective.

There are no clear guidelines as to how far to lower blood pressure in hypertensive encephalopathy, but it would seem prudent to avoid excessive falls in pressure. A target pressure of 160/110 has been recommended[2] at 24 h. Should the blood pressure fall too far, a head-down tilt of 30% may be all that is required; if a precipitous fall in pressure is accompanied by a slow heart rate, atropine should be given. For the reasons discussed under the management of uncomplicated MHT, it is probably unwise to attempt full control of blood pressure in the first week of treatment.

MANAGEMENT OF OTHER HYPERTENSIVE EMERGENCIES

Although other hypertensive emergencies are only occasionally associated with MHT, the principles of management are similar, and it may be useful to consider the following hypertensive emergencies.

Hypertension during myocardial infarction

A small increase in blood pressure is said to occur in up to 40% of cases of infarct[86]; very occasionally diastolic pressure may exceed 120 mmHg. The exact mechanism is unknown, but the rise in pressure may be mediated by high levels of circulating catecholamines. A cardiogenic reflex initiated by the release of serotonin from aggregating platelets in the proximal left coronary circulation has also been proposed[87] as the mechanism. Therapy should consist of relief of pain, and treatment of heart failure if it is present. When hypertension is severe, the addition of an intravenous vasodilator such as nitroglycerin, which dilates collateral blood vessels and may help to perfuse ischaemic myocardium, has been recommended[82]. For milder degrees of hypertension, a β-blocker, would seem a logical choice, following the recent demonstration that β-blockers given early in the course of myocardial infarction will not only lower blood pressure but also reduce in-hospital mortality[88].

Hypertension with acute stroke

Regrettably there are still no useful data to indicate how best to manage increased blood pressure in the presence of an acute stroke[2]. Special considerations in the hypertensive stroke patient are that blood pressure is often labile and may fall spontaneously, and also that the autoregulatory response is lost locally, causing cerebral blood flow to the ischaemic area to become pressure-dependent (Figure 2.3(d)).

There is the additional risk of vasospasm in patients with subarachnoid haemorrhage. Moreover, as already discussed, it can be difficult to distinguish between cerebral haemorrhage with severe hypertension and hypertensive encephalopathy.

It would seem sensible under the circumstances to withhold anti-hypertensive drugs for at least 24–48 hours if diastolic pressure is less than 120 mmHg. Treatment should then be initiated cautiously with either a thiazide diuretic or a β-blocker. If diastolic pressure is greater than 120 mmHg initially, the correct course of action is unclear, although a single oral dose of atenolol 50 mg or nifedipine retard 20 mg would seem reasonable in the first instance. Recourse to intravenous therapy may be necessary for the unconscious stroke patient.

The decision to treat and the choice of treatment would be made easier if the underlying pathology were known to be haemorrhage rather than infarction, since patients with haemorrhage are likely to bleed again if hypertension is uncontrolled, whereas the dangers of reducing blood pressure too quickly may be greater in the presence of infarction. Unfortunately, even this knowledge is usually denied, since few stroke patients can be given immediate access to a CT scanner. For all of these reasons, the management of hypertension in the setting of acute stroke remains a difficult problem for the general physician.

Phaeochromocytoma

The diagnosis of most cases of phaeochromocytoma can be confirmed by measurement of plasma or urinary catecholamines and the tumour can be localized by ultrasound or CT scan. α-Blockade should be established pre-operatively and the maximum tolerated dose of oral phenoxybenzamine should be given, even if hypertension is not present[89]. The starting dose is 10 mg daily and the dose range is 20–80 mg daily. Propranolol is indicated if there is persistent tachycardia or angina but it should never be prescribed before the phenoxy-benzamine, since unopposed α-vasoconstriction can further elevate blood pressure. In practice, it is probably safe to start both drugs simultaneously if both are required. Labetalol, a combined α- and β-blocker, has also been used successfully in phaeochromocytoma[90], but since it has less potent α-blocking than β-blocking properties, and since it is not possible to titrate α- and β-effects separately with this drug, it is not widely recommended for this purpose.

Phaeochromocytoma may occasionally present as a hypertensive emergency. An important clue to this diagnosis is the occurrence of severe hypertension in a patient who otherwise appears shocked, with pale, clammy extremities. Abdominal pain[91] or cardiac failure[92] may also be present. The drug of choice is phentolamine 5 mg by i.v. bolus, followed by further injections of 5 mg every few minutes to a total of 20 mg or until systemic vasoconstriction is relieved. A central line is recommended to monitor volume. Since the effect of phentolamine is transient, it may be necessary to maintain blood-pressure control by infusion at 1 mg/min until treatment with oral phenoxybenzamine can be established. Intravenous nitroprusside is also effective in controlling hypertension associated with increased circulating catecholamines[93] and may be preferable to phentolamine which is more likely to cause side-effects (Table 2.3). In addition, intravenous propranolol 1–10 mg or lignocaine 1–3 mg/kg may be required to correct arrhythmias. If therapy is prompt and appropriate, it should be possible to proceed to elective surgery at a later date.

Scleroderma renal crisis

Progressive systemic sclerosis may not infrequently be complicated by malignant hypertension and rapidly progressive renal failure; if it is untreated the outcome is invariably fatal. Patients with a short history and rapid increase in skin thickening are more likely to develop this complication[94]. The diagnosis is established by renal biopsy or by skin biopsy. It has been claimed that infusion of plasma[95] and/or use of converting enzyme inhibitors[95–97] may have a particular role to play in management; the evidence is, however, slight and it seems more likely that rigorous control of blood pressure by whatever means, together with dialysis if required, offers the best chance of renal recovery and survival[98–100]. Early bilateral nephrectomy, which was recommended previously[101], should certainly now be considered only when hypertension is resistant to medical therapy, since recovery of renal function may occur even after several months of dialysis[98–102].

Aortic dissection

Approximately two-thirds of patients with dissecting aneurysms of the aorta are severely hypertensive, and urgent reduction of blood pressure is required in these[103]. These measures should not delay surgery for acute dissections of the ascending aorta, but may be the treatment of choice when the lesion is confined to the descending aorta, since medical therapy is as good as surgery in such patients[104].

The ideal drug is one that reduces both blood pressure and ejection velocity (the velocity with which the contracting left ventricle ejects blood) and trimethaphan, a short-acting ganglion blocker, has traditionally been recommended[103]. In practice, however, most cardio-thoracic surgeons prefer intravenous nitroprusside for reducing blood pressure, with intravenous propranolol to reduce ejection velocity. The dose of propranolol is 1 mg initially followed by increments of 1 mg every 5 minutes until a heart rate of 50–60 per minute is achieved or a total dose of 10 mg has been given. The aim of therapy is to reduce systolic blood pressure to about 100 mmHg providing this can be tolerated by the patient. If long-term medical treatment is chosen, oral antihypertensives should be started after 48–72 hours with a view to maintaining systolic pressure in the range 100–130 mmHg[104].

SURVIVAL

In 1939, Keith et al.[105] published life tables showing that five-year survival in untreated patients with MHT was as low as 1%. Similar findings were reported among untreated patients from the U.K.[13]. With the advent and development of effective antihypertensive drug therapy[106], and more recently the introduction and increasing availability of renal dialysis and transplantation, the prognosis of MHT has improved such that in 1986 a five-year survival of at least 75% can be expected (Figure 2.5)[4]. Recently published data from other centres including Goteborg[3], Melbourne[5], and Leicester[6] support this view. All authors agree that the single most important predictor of outcome in MHT is the degree of renal impairment at initial presentation, and it seems likely that differences in the proportion of

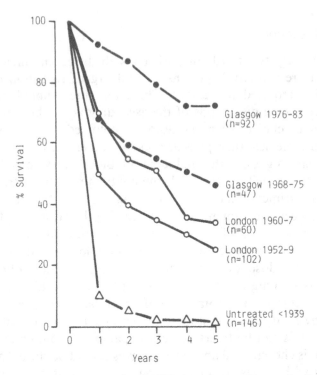

FIGURE 2.5   Five-year survival in MHT showing a progressive improvement in outcome with time. The untreated survival curve is from Keith *et
al.*[105], the London data from Breckenridge *et al.*[106] and the Glasgow data
from Isles *et al.*[4]

patients with impaired renal function will account for many of the
remaining 'discrepancies' in their results. Survival of patients with
renal function that is normal or only mildly impaired may be little
different from that of non-malignant hypertensives matched for age,
sex and pressure[4].

Two important exceptions to this encouraging trend are the studies
from Africa. In Johannesburg, only 75% of urban Blacks with MHT
survived to leave hospital. The long-term prognosis of these patients is
not known, since all survivors defaulted during follow-up[7]. A similarly
disappointing outcome has been reported from Kenya[61]. How much
this reflects inadequate facilities or the inability of poorly educated

people to grasp the concept of chronic illness is not clear. Irrespective of the cause, it is likely that MHT will remain for some time a greater medical and social problem in the developing world than it is in the West.

EFFECT OF TREATMENT ON RETINOPATHY AND VISION

The risk of precipitating or exacerbating visual loss when blood pressure is lowered too quickly in patients with MHT has already been discussed. In most patients with MHT, the retinal lesions clear and vision improves with effective treatment[64]. Even the most severe retinopathy can resolve given time and adequate control of blood pressure. Although a fully formed macular star may take a year to disappear (Figure 2.6(a), (b)), less severe retinopathy clears over a period of 3–6 months (Figure 2.6(c)). Not every fundus returns completely to normal, however, and three late changes may occasionally be seen: optic atrophy (Figure 2.6(d)), pipe-stem sclerosis of the retinal arterioles (Figure 2.6(d)) and Elschnig's spots (areas of black pigment representing small choroidal infarcts), (Figure 2.6(e)). Patients who present with severe maculopathy, or who develop optic atrophy, may have residual visual impairment, but otherwise, and in the great majority of patients, the prognosis for vision is excellent.

EFFECT OF TREATMENT ON RENAL FUNCTION

The initial management of patients with MHT and impaired renal function has been considered, as has the importance of the serum creatinine concentration in determining long-term survival. In the following section, the renal outcome of patients with MHT will be analysed in more detail.

It is useful to consider short-term changes in renal function and long-term renal outcome separately. Lawton[107] studied the short-term course of renal function in malignant hypertensives with renal insufficiency and concluded that when blood pressure is controlled initially, renal function will stabilize in 10% of cases, deteriorate progressively in 30%, and deteriorate transiently before improving in the remainder. Lawton also showed that the last group can usually be

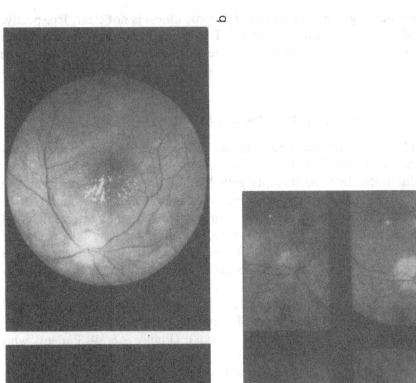

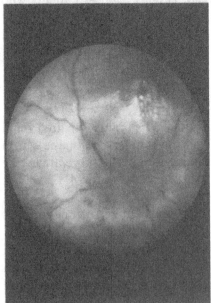

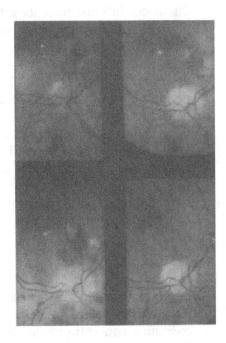

a

b

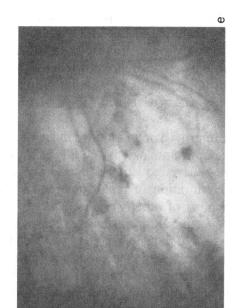

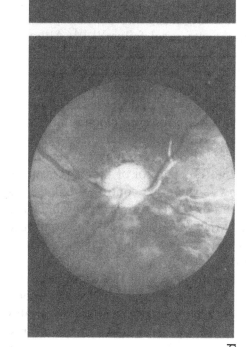

FIGURE 2.6 (a) and (b) Fundal appearances of a 15-year-old girl with MHT, taken at presentation (a) and after 9 months of treatment (b). Papilloedema had resolved completely by this time, but the macular star was still present. (c) Resolution of fundal changes in a less severe case. Moving from top left in a clockwise direction, these photographs were taken 3, 5, 8 and 16 weeks after presentation. By 16 weeks the papilloedema and most of the haemorrhage and soft exudate had disappeared, leaving only a small trace of hard exudate. (d) Optic atrophy and pipe-stem sclerosis of the retinal arterioles. 2 years after successful treatment for MHT. (e) Choroidal infarcts (Elschnig's spots) are another late feature occasionally seen in MHT. The photograph is an enlarged view of the fundus with the optic disc at top right.

identified after 2 weeks of antihypertensive therapy and that, in the short term, patients with primary renal parenchymal disease did not have a worse prognosis than those without primary renal disease. These findings are entirely consistent with current knowledge regarding the benefits of treatment to the hypertensive vascular lesions in the kidney and the possible adverse effects of reducing renal perfusion pressure.

Whether renal function can be improved or maintained by treatment in the long term is perhaps more important. Woods and Blythe[108] were among the first to show that aggressive reduction of blood pressure did not necessarily result in deterioration of renal function. These findings were confirmed by a number of other workers, [109,110]. In the series reported by Pohl et al.[110], effective antihypertensive therapy was shown to improve the renal function of patients who had survived for 6 months, whose initial creatinine clearance was greater than 8 ml/min and in whom there was no instrinsic progressive renal disease. The improvement in renal function was maintained during 43 months follow-up.

More recent still has been the wider recognition of the syndrome of malignant hypertension with acute renal failure[111-114]. Although uncommon, the diagnosis should be considered in all patients with MHT and renal failure, especially if oliguric, since the prospects for improvement of renal function are good. Characteristic features of this syndrome include normal-sized kidneys on high-dose urography, and marked vascular changes with well-preserved glomeruli on renal biopsy. Intimal proliferation and oedema of the small renal arteries may lead to acute tubular necrosis that in turn may be responsible for the acute renal failure[114]. Rigorous control of blood pressure is essential. Peritoneal dialysis allows a smoother control of blood pressure than does haemodialysis, and may therefore be preferable when acute renal failure complicates MHT. Dialysis should be continued for a period of several months before it can be concluded that recovery of renal function will not occur.

Data from the Glasgow series may usefully illustrate all of the preceding points (Figures 2.7 and 2.8). The renal function of patients with an underlying renal cause for their hypertension almost invariably deteriorated during long-term follow-up, irrespective of blood-pressure control, such that all patients with glomerulonephritis and most with interstitial nephropathy had developed end-stage renal failure by the end of the study. It seems likely that deterioration of renal function in these patients simply represents the natural history of a progressive underlying disease. By contrast, renal function in MHT associated with renovascular disease deteriorated in 3 of 17 patients only (Figure 2.7). Overall survival in these patients was no better, however, than in the renal parenchymal group, presumably as a result of widespread atheromatous disease affecting the coronary and cerebral circulation as well as the renal circulation.

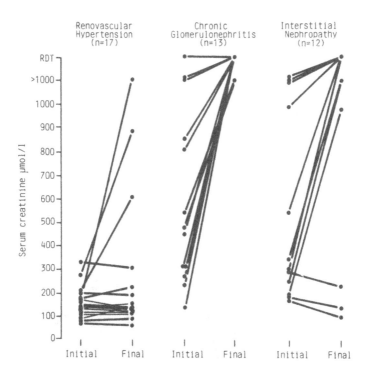

FIGURE 2.7 Changes in renal function during follow-up of MHT in patients with renovascular disease, chronic glomerulonephritis and interstial nephropathy. The values shown are initial and final serum creatinine concentration. At least 1 year separates each pair of measurements except for cases where rapidly advancing renal failure led to a patient's death. These data therefore represent long-term rather than short-term changes in renal function.

69

The renal outcome of patients considered to have the malignant phase of essential hypertension is shown in Figure 2.8, in which there appear to be three groups of patients, each with a different renal prognosis. (1) Patients whose serum creatinine concentration is below 300 μmol at the time of presentation, most of whom do well with

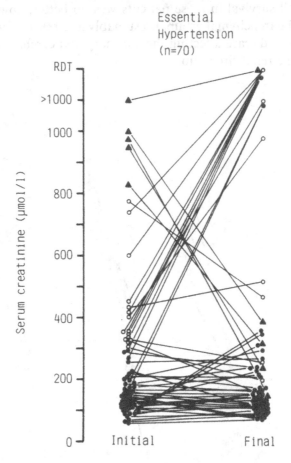

FIGURE 2.8   Changes in renal function during follow-up of patients with malignant phase of essential hypertension. Criteria for inclusion as per Figure 3.7. Solid circles represent patients whose serum creatinine was below 300μmol/l at time of presentation (n= 50). Open circles represent patients with chronic renal failure who did not require dialysis immediately (n=15). Solid triangles represent patients with syndrome of malignant hypertension and acute oliguric renal failure (n= 5).

effective antihypertensive therapy. (2) Patients who present with chronic renal failure but do not require dialysis immediately. These patients are less likely to maintain or recover renal function except possibly in the short term[107] and progression to end-stage renal failure is common. (3) A small group with acute renal failure. These patients rarely give a past history of renal impairment. The only certain way to establish the diagnosis, and to exclude underlying renal disease, is by renal biopsy. In the Glasgow series, 5 of 139 patients with MHT presented with acute renal failure, and in 4 of these renal function improved significantly following a period of dialysis and meticulous blood pressure control. These findings imply that in malignant essential hypertension, irreversible renal damage will usually have occurred by the time the serum creatinine concentration exceeds 300 μmol unless acute renal failure is superimposed.

CONCLUSION

Although much has been achieved in recent years, much remains to be done, The relative importance of genetic and socioeconomic factors in the pathogenesis of malignant hypertension has still to be determined. So too has the reason why some patients with diastolic pressures greater than 130 mmHg enter the malignant phase while others do not. Not enough is known of the effects of different antihypertensive drugs on cerebral blood flow at different arterial pressures to allow a confident conclusion concerning the ideal rate of reduction of blood pressure in patients who have this disease. It is also unclear whether further improvements in survival for patients with significant renal impairment can be expected. The problem in the U.K. is that doctors no longer see enough MHT, even in renal units, to answer these questions. The burden of work must then inevitably fall on units that do see it, probably those in Africa and South America[2].

Acknowledgements

I should like to thank Drs J. D. Briggs, J. J. Brown, J. Dougall, J. L. Jay, R. M. Isles, A. F. Lever, G. Lindop, I. C. Macdougall, G. T.

McInnes and J. McLenachan for their helpful comments during the preparation of this paper, and also to acknowledge Miss Angela McKay who typed the script.

References

1. Kincaid-Smith, P. (1985). What has happened to malignant hypertension? In Bulpitt, C. J. (ed). *Handbook of Hypertension, Vol 6, Epidemiology of Hypertension*, pp. 225–65. (Amsterdam: Elsevier)
2. Ledingham, J. G. G. (1983). Management of hypertensive crises. *Hypertension*, **5** (Suppl. III), 114–19
3. Gudbrandsson, T., Hansson, L., Herlitz, H. and Andren, L. (1979). Malignant hypertension – improving prognosis in a rare disease. *Acta Med, Scand.*, **206**, 495–9.
4. Isles, C. G., Lim, K. G., Boulton-Jones, M., Cameron, H., Lever, A. F., Murray, G. and Robertson, J. W. K. (1985). Factors influencing outcome in malignant hypertension. *J. Hypertension*, **3**, (Suppl. 3), S405–7
5. Yu, S. H., Whitworth, J. A. and Kincaid-Smith, P. S. (1986). Malignant hypertension: etiology and outcome in eighty-three patients. *Clin. Exp. Hypertension*, **A8**, 1211–30
6. Bing, R. F., Heagerty, A. M., Russell, G. I., Swales, J. D. and Thurston, H. (1986). Prognosis in malignant hypertension. *J. Hypertension*, **4** (Suppl. 6), S42–S44
7. Jhetam, D., Dansey, R., Morar, C., and Milne, F. J. (1982). The malignant phase of essential hypertension in Johannesburg blacks. *S. Afr. Med. J.*, **61**, 899–902
8. World Health Organisation (1978). Arterial hypertension. *WHO Tech. Rep. Ser.*, **628**, 57
9. Pickering, G. W. (1968). *High blood pressure.* (London: Churchill)
10. Reubi, F. (1974). Malignant hypertension. *Clin. Nephrol.*, **2**, 211–14
11. Kincaid-Smith, P. (1981). Understanding malignant hypertension. *Austr. N.Z. J. Med.*, **11**, (Suppl. 1), 64–8
12. Schottstaedt, M. F. and Sokolow, M. (1953). The natural history and course of hypertension with papilloedema (malignant hypertension). *Am. Heart. J.*, **45**, 331–62
13. Kincaid-Smith, P., McMichael, J. and Murphy E. A. (1958). The clinical course and pathology of hypertension with papilloedema (malignant hypertension). *Q. J. Med.*, **27**, 117–53
14. Gifford, R. W. (1983). Management and treatment of essential hypertension including malignant hypertension and emergencies. In Genest, J., Kuchel, O., Hamet, P., and Cantin, M. (Eds). *Hypertension: physiopathology and treatment, 2nd Edn.*, pp. 1127–70. (New York: McGraw-Hill)
15. Brown, J. J., Davies, D. L., Lever, A. F., and Robertson, J. I. S. (1966). Plasma renin concentration in human hypertension III: renin in relation to complications of hypertension. *Br. Med. J.*, **1**, 505–8
16. McLeod, D., Marshall, J. and Kohner, E. M. (1980). Role of axoplasmic transport in the pathophysiology of ischaemic disc swelling. *Br. J. Ophthalmol.*, **64**, 247–61

17. Wrong, O. (1986). Retinal changes in malignant/accelerated hypertension. *Br. Med. J.*, **1**, 483
18. McGregor, E., Isles, C. G., Jay, J. L., Lever, A. F. and Murray, G. D. (1986). Retinal changes in malignant hypertension. *Br. Med. J.*, **1**, 233–4
19. Ahmed, M. E. K., Walker, J. M., Beevers, D. G. and Beevers, M. (1986). Lack of difference between malignant and accelerated hypertension. *Br. Med. J.*, **1**, 235–7
20. Lindop, G. (1985). Blood vessels and lymphatics. In Anderson, J. R. (Ed.) *Muir's textbook of pathology, 12th Edn.*, Chap. 14. (Edinburgh: Edward Arnold)
21. Beilin, L. J. and Goldby, F. S. (1977). High arterial pressure versus humoral factors in the pathogenesis of vascular lesions of malignant hypertension: the case for pressure alone. *Clin. Sci.*, **52**, 111–13
22. Gudbrandsson, T., Hansson L., Herlitz, H., Lindholm L. and Nilsson L. A. (1981). Immunological changes in patients with previous malignant essential hypertension. *Lancet*, **1**, 406–8
23. Gavras, H., Oliver, N., Aitchison, J., Begg, C., Briggs, J. D., Brown, J. J., Horton, P. W., Lee, F., Lever, A. F., Prentice, C. R. M. and Robertson, J. I. S. (1975). Abnormalities of coagulation and the development of malignant phase hypertension. *Kidney Int.*, **8**, S252–61
24. Isles, C. G., Lowe, G. D. O., Rankin, B. M., Forbes, C. D., Lucie, N., Lever, A. F. and Kennedy, A. C. (1984). Abnormal haemostasis and blood viscosity in malignant hypertension. *Thromb. Haemostas.*, **52**, 253–5
25. Isles, C. G., Brown, J. J., Cumming, A. M. M., Lever, A. F., McAreavey, D., Robertson, J. I. S., Hawthorne, V. M., Stewart, G. M., Robertson, J. W. K. and Wapshaw, J. (1979). Excess smoking in malignant phase hypertension. *Br. Med. J.*, **1**, 579–81
26. Bloxham, C. A., Beevers, D. G. and Walker, J. M. (1979). Malignant hypertension and cigarette smoking. *Br. Med. J.*, **1**, 581–3
27. Harris, P. W. R. (1969). Malignant hypertension associated with oral contraceptives. *Lancet*, **2**, 466–7
28. Giese, J. (1976). The renin-angiotensin system and the pathogenesis of vascular disease in malignant hypertension. *Clin. Sci.*, **51**, 19s–21s
29. Mohring, J. (1977). High arterial pressure versus humoral factors in the pathogenesis of vascular lesions of malignant hypertension: the case for humoral factors as well as pressure. *Clin Sci.*, **52**, 113–17
30. Geise, J. (1964). Acute hypertensive vascular disease, 2. Studies on vascular reaction patterns and permeability changes by means of vital microscopy and celloidal tracer technique. *Acta Pathol. Microbiol. Scand*, **62**, 497–515
31. Ross, R. and Glomsett, J. A. (1973). Atherosclerosis and the arterial smooth muscle cell: proliferation of smooth muscle is a key event in the genesis of lesions of atherosclerosis. *Science*, **180**, 1332–9
32. Linton, A. L., Gavras, H., Gleadle, R. I., Hutchison, H. E., Lawson, D. H., Lever, A. F., MacAdam, R. F., McNicol, G. P. and Robertson, J. I. S. (1969). Microangiopathic haemolytic anaemia and the pathogenesis of malignant hypertension. *Lancet*, **1**, 1277–82
33. Robertson, J. I. S. (1986). Hypertension in the elderly. *Triangle*, **25**, 19–23
34. Lee, T. H and Alderman, M. H. (1978). Malignant hypertension: declining mortality rate in New York city, 1958–1974. *N.Y. State J. Med.*, **78**, 1389–91

35. Davis, B. A., Crook, J. E., Vestal, R. E. and Oates, J. A. (1979). Prevalence of renovascular hypertension in patients with grade III or IV hypertensive retinopathy. *N. Engl. J. Med.*, **301**, 1273–6

36. Ferris, J. B., Beevers, D. G., Brown, J. J., Davies, D. L., Fraser, R., Lever, A. F., Mason, P., Neville, A. M., Robertson, J. I. S. (1978). Clinical, biochemical and pathological features of low-renin (primary) hyperaldosteronism. *Am. Heart J.*, **95**, 375–88

37. Murphy, B. F., Whitworth, J. A and Kincaid-Smith, P. (1985). Malignant hypertension due to an aldosterone producing adrenal adenoma. *Clin. Exp. Hypertension*, **A7**, 939–50

38. Gold, C. H., Isaacson, C., and Levin, J. (1982). The pathological basis of end stage renal disease in blacks. *S. Afr. Med. J.*, **61**, 263–5

39. Sinclair, A. M., Isles, C. G., Brown, I., Cameron, H., Murray, G. D., Robertson, J. W. K. and Wapshaw, J. (1987). Secondary hypertension in a blood pressure clinic. *Arch. Intern. Med.*, **147**, 1289–93

40. Seltzer, C. C. (1974). Effect of smoking on blood pressure. *Am. Heart. J.*, **87**, 558–64

41. Freestone, S. and Ramsay, L. E. (1982). Effect of coffee and cigarette smoking on the blood pressure of untreated and diuretic-treated hypertensive patients. *Am. J. Med.*, **73**, 348–53

42. MRC Working Party. (1985). Medical Research Council Trial of treatment of mild hypertension: principal results. *Br. Med. J.*, **2**, 97–104

43. Elliott, J. M. and Simpson, F. O. (1980). Cigarettes and accelerated hypertension. *N.Z. Med. J.*, **91**, 447–9

44. Tuomilehto, J., Elo, J. and Nissmen, A. (1982). Smoking among patients with malignant hypertension. *Br. Med. J.*, **1**, 1086

45. Royal College of Physicians (1977). *Smoking or health?* Third Report. (London: Pitman Medical)

46. Zacherle, B. J. and Richardson, J. A. (1972). Irreversible renal failure secondary to hypertension induced by oral contraceptives. *Ann. Intern. Med.*, **77**, 83–5

47. Dunn, F. G., Jones, J. V. and Fife, R. (1975). Malignant hypertension associated with use of oral contraceptives. *Br. Heart J.*, **37**, 336–8

48. Zech, P., Rifle, G., Lindner, A., Sassard, J., Blanc-Brunat, N. and Traeger, J. (1975). Malignant hypertension with irreversible renal failure due to oral contraceptives. *Br. Med. J.*, **4**, 326–7

49. Saint Hillier, Y., Baumont, N., Colomb, H., Pageaut, G. and Perol, C. (1977). Hypertension arterielle maligne et contraceptifs oraux. *J. Urol. Nephrol.* (Paris), **83**, 673–9

50. Hodsman, G. P., Robertson, J. I. S., Semple, P. F. and MacKay, A. (1982). Malignant hypertension and oral contraceptives: four cases, with two due to the 30μg oestrogen pill. *Eur. Heart J.*, **3**, 255–9

51. Pettiti, D. B. and Klatsky, A. L. (1983). Malignant hypertension in women aged 15–44 years and its relation to cigarette smoking and oral contraceptives. *Am. J. Cardiol.*, **52**, 297–8

52. Lim, K. G., Isles, C. G., Hodsman, G. P., Lever, A. F. and Robertson, J. W. K. (1987). Malignant hypertension in women of childbearing age and its relation to the oral contraceptive pill. *Br. Med. J.*, **1**, 1057–9

53. Mammen, E. F. (1982). Oral contraceptives and blood coagulation: a critical review. *Am. J. Obstet. Gynaecol.*, **142**, 781–90

54. Golbus, S. M., Swerdlin, A. R., Mitas, J. A., Rowley, W. R., James, D. R. (1979). Renal artery thrombosis in a young woman taking oral contraceptives. *Ann. Intern. Med.,* **90,** 939–40
55. Boyd, W. N., Burden, R. P. and Aber, G. M. (1975). Intrarenal vascular changes in patients receiving oestrogen containing compounds – a clinical, histological and angiographic study. *Q. J. Med.,* **44,** 415–31
56. Sleight, P. (1984). Hypertension. In Weatherall, D. J., Ledingham, J. G. G. and Warrell, D. A. (Eds.) *Oxford Textbook of Medicine, Vol. 2,* pp. 258–78 (Oxford: Oxford University Press)
57. Ying, C. Y., Tifft, C. P., Gavras, H. and Chobanian, A. V. (1984). Renal revascularisation in the azotaemic hypertensive patient resistant to therapy. *N. Engl. J. Med.* **311,** 1070–5
58. Gudbrandsson, T., Swertsson, R., Herlitz, H. and Hansson, L. (1982). Cardiac involvement in hypertension: a non invasive study of patients with previous malignant hypertension and 'benign' hypertension. *Eur. Heart J.,* **3,** 246–54
59. Shapiro, L. M., MacKinnon, J. and Beevers, D. G. (1981). Echocardiographic features of malignant hypertension. *Br. Heart J.,* **46,** 374–9
60. Healton, E. B., Brust, J. C., Feinfield, D. A. and Thomson, G. E. (1982). Hypertensive encephalopathy and the neurological manifestations of malignant hypertension. *Neurology,* **32,** 127–32
61. Bahemuka, M. (1985). Malignant hypertension: a review of the neurological features in 34 consecutive patients. *E. Afr. Med. J.,* **62,** 560–5
62. Barcenas, C. G., Gonzales-Molina, M., and Hull, A. R. (1978). Association between acute pancreatitis and malignant hypertension with renal failure. *Arch. Intern. Med.* **138,** 1254–6
63. Padfield, P. L. (1975). Malignant hypertension presenting with an acute abdomen. *Br. Med. J.,* **3,** 353–4
64. Dollery, C. T. (1983). Hypertensive retinopathy. In Genest, J., Kuchel, O., Hamet, P. and Cantin, M. (Eds.) *Hypertension: Physiopathology and Treatment, 2nd Edn.,* pp. 723–32. (Toronto: MacGraw-Hill)
65. Breslin, D. J., Ray, M. D., Gifford, R. W., Fairbairn, J. F. and Kearns, T. P. (1966). Prognostic importance of ophthalmoscopic findings in essential hypertension. *J. Am. Med. Assoc.,* **195,** 335–8
66. Pears, M. A. and Pickering, G. W. (1960). Changes in the fundus oculi after haemorrhage. *Q. J. Med,* **29,** 153–80
67. Ballantyne, A. J. and Michaelson, I. C. (1962). Disorders of blood and blood forming organs. *Textbook of the Fundus and Eye,* pp. 216–25. (Edinburgh: Livingstone)
68. Knowler, W. C., Bennett, P. H. and Ballintine, E. J. (1980). Increased incidence of retinopathy in diabetics with elevated blood pressure. *N. Engl. J. Med.,* **302,** 645–50
69. Strandgaard, S. and Paulson, O. B. (1984). Cerebral autoregulation. *Stroke,* **15,** 413–16
70. Graham, D. I., Lee, W. R., Cumming, A. M. M., Robertson, J. I. S. and Jones, J. V. (1983). Hypertension and the intracranial and intraoccular circulations: effects of antihypertensive treatment. In Robertson, J. I. S. (Ed.) *Handbook of Hypertension, Vol. Clinical Aspects of Essential Hypertension,* pp. 174–201. (Amsterdam: Elsevier)

71. Graham, D. I. (1975). Ischaemic brain damage of cerebral perfusion failure type following treatment of severe hypertension: a report of two cases. *Br. Med. J.,* **2,** 739
72. Ledingham, J. G. G. and Rajagopalan, B. (1979). Cerebral complications in the treatment of accelerated hypertension. *Q. J. Med.,* **48,** 25–41
73. Cove, D. H., Seddon, M., Fletcher, R. F. and Dukes, D. C. (1979). Blindness after treatment for malignant hypertension. *Br. Med. J.,* **2,** 245–6
74. Hulse, J. A., Taylor, D. S. I. and Dillon, M. J. (1979). Blindness and paraplegia in severe childhood hypertension. *Lancet,* **2,** 553–6
75. Isles, C. G., Johnston, A. O. C. and Milne, F. J. (1986). Slow release Nifedipine and Atenolol as initial treatment in blacks with malignant hypertension. *Br. J. Clin, Pharmacol.,* **21,** 377–83
76. Bannan, L. P. and Beevers, D. G. (1981). Emergency treatment of high blood pressure with oral Atenolol. *Br. Med. J.,* **1,** 1757–8
77. Bertel, P., Conen, D., Radu, E. W., Muller, J., Lang, C. and Dubach, U. C. (1983). Nifedipine in hypertensive emergencies. *Br. Med. J.,* **1,** 19–21
78. Merrill, J. P. (1962). Hypertensive vascular disease. In Harrison, T. R., Resnik, W. R., Wintrobe, M. M., Thorn, G. W., Adams, R. D. and Bennett, I. L. (Eds.) *Principles of Internal Medicine,* p. 1359. (New York: McGraw-Hill).
79. Mailloux, L. U., Mossey, R. T., Susin, M. and Teichberg, S. (1981). Does treatment of hypertension prevent renal failure? *Clin. Exp. Dial. Apher.,* **5,** 197–212
80. Vidt, D. G., Bravo, E. L. and Fouad, F. M. (1982). Drug therapy: Captopril. *N. Engl. J. Med.,* **306,** 214–8
81. Abe, I., Kawasaki, T., Kawazoe, N. and Omae, T. (1983). Acute electrocardiographic effects of captopril in the initial treatment of malignant or severe hypertension. *Am. Heart J.,* **106,** 558–62
82. Vidt, D. G. and Gifford, R. W. (1984). A compendium for the treatment of hypertensive emergencies. *Cleve. Clin. Q.,* **51,** 421–30
83. Dinsdale, H. B. (1982). Hypertensive encephalopathy. *Stroke,* **13,** 717–19
84. Palmer, R. F. and Lasseter, K. C. (1975). Sodium nitroprusside. *N. Engl. J. Med.,* **292,** 294–7
85. Cummings, A. M. M., Brown, J. J., Fraser, R., Lever, A. F., Morton, J. J., Richards, D. A. and Robertson, J. I. S. (1979). Blood pressure reduction by incremental infusion of labetalol in patients with severe hypertension. *Br. J. Clin. Pharmacol.,* **8,** 359–64
86. Dunn, F. G. (1983). Hypertension and myocardial infarction. *J. Am. Coll. Cardiol.,* **1,** 528–32
87. Dye, L. E., Urthaler, F., MacLean, W. A. H., Russell, R. O., Rackley, C. E. and James, T. N. (1978). New arterial hypertension during myocardial infarction. *South. Med. J.,* **71,** 289–92
88. ISIS-1 (First international study of infarct survival) Collaborative group (1986). Randomised trial of intravenous atenolol among 16,027 cases of suspected acute myocardial infarction: ISIS-1. *Lancet,* **2,** 57–66
89. Ball, S. G. (1984). Phaeochromocytoma. In Robertson, J. I. S. (Ed.) *Handbook of Hypertension, Vol. II, Clinical Aspects of Secondary Hypertension,* pp. 238–75 (Amsterdam: Elsevier)
90. Agabiti-Rosei, E., Brown, J. J., Lever, A. F., Morton, J. J., Robertson, A. M., Robertson, J. I. S. and Trust, P. M. (1976). Treatment of phaeochromocytoma

and of clonidine withdrawal hypertension with labetalol. *Br. J. Clin. Pharmacol.,* **3,** (Suppl. 3), 809–15

91. Jones, D. J. and Durning, P. (1985). Phaeochromocytoma presenting as an acute abdomen: report of two cases. *Br. Med. J.,* **2,** 1267–8

92. Shapiro, L. M., Trethowan, N. and Singh, S. P. (1982). Normotensive cardiomyopathy and malignant hypertension in phaeochromocytoma. *Postgrad. Med. J.,* **58,** 110–11

93. Editorial (1978). Controlled intravascular nitroprusside treatment. *Br. Med. J.,* **2,** 784–5

94. Steen, V. D., Medsger, T. A., Osial, T. A., Ziegler, G. L., Shapiro, A. P. and Rodnan, G. P. (1984). Factors predicting development of renal involvement in progressive systemic sclerosis. *Am. J. Med.,* **76,** 779–86

95. Ponticelli, C., Ambroso, G., Graziani, G., Rossi, E. (1980). Reversible acute renal failure in diffuse scleroderma. *Clin. Nephrol.,* **13,** 293–5

96. Zawada, E. T., Clements, P. J., Furst, D. A., Bloomer, A., Paulus, H. E and Maxwell, M. H. (1981). Clinical course of patients with scleroderma renal crisis treated with Captopril. *Nephron,* **27,** 74–8

97. Chapman, P. J., Pascoe, M. D. and Van Zyl-Smit, R. (1986). Successful use of Captopril in the treatment of scleroderma renal crisis. *Clin. Nephrol,* **26,** 106–8

98. Mitnick, P. D. and Feig, P. U. (1978). Control of hypertension and reversal of renal failure in scleroderma. *N. Engl. J. Med.,* **299,** 871–2

99. Simon, N. M., Graham, M. B., Kyser, F. A. and Gashti, E. N. (1979). Resolution of renal failure with malignant hypertension in scleroderma. *Am. J. Med.,* **67,** 533–9

100. Traub, Y. M., Shapiro, A. P., Osial, T. A., Rodnan, G. P., Medsger, T. A., Leb, D. E. and Christy, W. C. (1981). Response of patients with renal involvement by progressive systemic sclerosis to antihypertensive therapy. *Clin. Sci.,* **61,** 395s–8s

101. Richardson, J. A. (1973). Haemodialysis and kidney transplantation for renal failure from scleroderma. *Arthritis Rheum.,* **16,** 265–71

102. Lam, M., Ricanati, E. S., Khan, M. A. *et al.* (1978). Reversal of severe renal failure in systemic sclerosis. *Ann. Intern. Med.,* **89,** 642–3

103. Doroghazi, R. M., Slater, E. E. and De Sanctis, R. W. (1981). Medical therapy for aortic dissections. *J. Cardiovasc. Med.,* **6,** 187–98

104. Najafi, H. (1983). Aortic dissection. In Sabiston, D. C. and Spencer, F. C. (Eds.) *Surgery of the Chest,* 4th Edn., pp. 956–67. (Philadelphia: W. B. Saunders)

105. Keith, N. M., Wagener, H. P. and Barker, N. W. (1939). Some different types of essential hypertension: their course and prognoses. *Am. J. Med. Sci.,* **197,** 332–43

106. Breckenridge, A., Dollery, C. T. and Parry, E. H. O. (1970). Prognosis of treated hypertension: changes in life expectancy and causes of death between 1952 and 1967. *Q. J. Med.,* **39,** 411–29

107. Lawton, W. J. (1982). The short term course of renal function in malignant hypertensives with renal insufficiency. *Clin. Nephrol.,* **17,** 277–83

108. Woods, J. W. and Blythe, W. B. (1967). Management of malignant hypertension complicated by renal insufficiency. *N. Engl. J. Med.,* **277,** 57–61

109. Mroczek, W. J., Davidov, M., Gavrilovich, L. and Finnerty, F. A. (1969). The value of aggressive therapy in the hypertensive patient with azotaemia. *Circulation,* **40,** 893–904

110. Pohl, J. E. F., Thurston, H. and Swales, J. D. (1974). Hypertension with renal impairment: influence of intensive therapy. *Q. J. Med.*, **43**, 569–81
111. Sevitt, L. H., Evans, D. J. and Wrong, O. M. (1971). Acute oliguric renal failure due to accelerated (malignant) hypertension. *Q. J. Med.*, **40**, 127–44
112. Mamdani, B. H., Lim, V. S., Mahurkar, S. D., Katz, A. I. and Dunea, G. (1974). Recovery from prolonged renal failure in patients with accelerated hypertension. *N. Engl. J. Med.*, **291**, 1343–4
113. Cordingley, F. T., Jones, N. F., Wing, A. J. and Hilton, P. J. (1980). Reversible renal failure in malignant hypertension. *Clin. Nephrol.*, **14**, 98–103
114. Isles, C. G., McLay, A. and Boulton-Jones, J. M. (1984). Recovery in malignant hypertension presenting as acute renal failure. *Q. J. Med.*, **53**, 439–52

3
SURGICAL MANAGEMENT OF RENAL HYPERTENSION

J. A. MURIE and P. J. MORRIS

INTRODUCTION

The evaluation and management of renovascular hypertension has been a controversial issue for many years. Unfortunately, many relevant investigative and therapeutic techniques have been studied in a somewhat uncontrolled fashion, often involving patient populations that were unique to the investigating centres. Truly scientific comparisons of both methods of evaluation and management programmes have been relatively few. To this background has now been added a new investigative advance, digital subtraction angiography, and a new therapeutic advance, percutaneous transluminal angioplasty. These two developments, which have had a major influence in other areas of vascular surgery, have similarly had a major impact on the diagnosis and management of renovascular disease. Particular regard is paid to them in this volume, digital subtraction angiography in the present chapter and balloon angioplasty in Chapter 4.

Pathophysiology

Renovascular disease is the commonest cause of surgically curable hypertension. The prevalence of renovascular hypertension in the general hypertensive population is often said[1,2] to be about 1%, but estimates as low as 0.2%[3] and as high as 5%[4,5] have been suggested by others. Thornbury[6] has recently reviewed the literature and suggested 3% as an average current figure. This value is important when we come to consider the planning of investigation for putative renovascular hypertension.

Although renal insufficiency is not usually regarded as a typical presenting feature of renovascular hypertension, this may be due to the difficulty of distinguishing, on clinical grounds, patients with hypertension and renal failure due to renal artery stenosis from those with long-standing essential hypertension and nephrosclerosis, and from others with hypertension due to primary renal parenchymal disease. Severe atheromatous narrowing of the renal arteries is a bilateral phenomenon in over one-third of patients with renovascular hypertension[5] and renal artery stenosis (RAS) may be responsible for the elevation of blood pressure in almost 50% of those with renal insufficiency in association with refractory hypertension[7].

While moderate unilateral RAS may cause hypertension, major bilateral occlusive disease is required before renal failure occurs; and since atheroma is a chronologically progressive pathology, it would seem reasonable to view renovascular hypertension in association with renal insufficiency as representing the end-stage of the disease process. Indeed it has been shown that when renovascular hypertension is treated medically, a rise in serum creatinine and fall in glomerular filtration rate can be expected in nearly half the patients over a 28-month period[8]. In this same series, over 40% of patients experienced a reduction in renal function or loss of renal size that precipitated surgical intervention; a renal artery stenosis had progressed to total occlusion in 12%. Unfortunately, it is not yet possible to predict early which patients will exhibit such progressive disease.

TABLE 3.1 Underlying arterial pathology in 60 patients operated on for renovascular disease in Oxford

Pathology	No.	Per cent of total
Atheroma	50	83
Trauma	4	7
Fibromuscular dysplasia	3	5
Other	3	5

Several other pathologies may affect the calibre of the renal artery: these include fibromuscular dysplasia, trauma, embolic disease, Takayasu's disease and other arteritides. Although trauma has been the second commonest pathology underlying surgically corrected RAS in Oxford (Table 3.1), fibromuscular dysplasia, which may cause up to 20% of RAS cases[9], should in general be ranked second after atheroma. While atheroma generally affects the origin or proximal third of the main renal artery, giving rise to an eccentric or, less commonly, a concentric narrowing, often with post-stenotic dilatation (Figure 3.1), fibromuscular dysplasia tends to involve the middle or distal segments of the main artery and even the branch arteries. The incidence of bilateral involvement is greater than for atheroma, with bilateral lesions occurring in at least half of affected patients. The main pathological types of dysplasia are intimal fibroplasia, medial

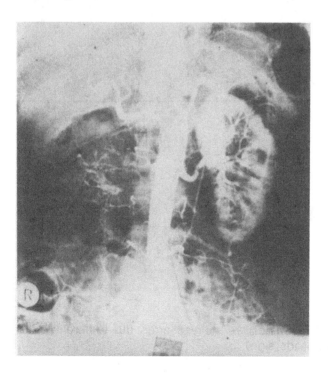

FIGURE 3.1 Atheromatous stenosis of the left renal artery. The right renal artery is thrombosed

81

fibroplasia, medial hyperplasia and perimedial fibroplasia[10]. Medial fibroplasia is the most commonly encountered dysplasia and gives rise to the classic 'string of beads' appearance on angiography (Figure 3.2). Other radiological appearances may include focal stenosis and medial dissection with fusiform dilatation[11].

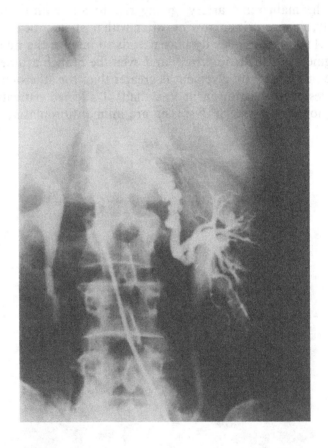

FIGURE 3.2   Stenosis of the renal artery due to fibromuscular dysplasia ('string of beads' sign)

Clinical features

The clinical features of renovascular hypertension have been assessed by the Cooperative Study of Renovascular Hypertension[12]. It is difficult to differentiate between renovascular and essential hypertension on clinical grounds. While there is recognition that certain features are found more commonly in one type than in the other, a considerable overlap exists and no single feature is unique to either disease.

The most distinguishing clinical feature is the presence of an abdominal or flank bruit, but, since essential hypertension is many times commoner than renovascular hypertension, such a bruit occurs in similar numbers in each group. The clinician should also be aware that the recognition of bruit using a simple stethoscope is fraught with problems. The Cooperative Study group recognized that such murmurs were much easier to hear in thin patients than in obese patients[12] and at other arterial sites, such as the carotid, high-grade stenoses have been shown to reduce blood flow to such an extent that audible turbulence is unlikely[13].

Although obesity is present in more than one-third of patients with essential hypertension, it is not particularly common in cases of renovascular hypertension. Twenty-three per cent of patients with essential hypertension entering the Cooperative Study had had known elevated blood pressure for over 10 years compared with only 11% of those with renovascular hypertension, and essential hypertension had in general been present for 1 year longer than renovascular hypertension. It is surprising that the biochemical features of aldosteronism were not more common in the renovascular group, since symptomatic RAS is frequently associated with increased activity of the renin–angiotensin system. Hypokalaemia occurred two or three times more often in renovascular than in essential hypertension, but was found in less than 20% of cases. Bacteriuria is also commoner in renovascular disease. It has been shown to occur in 18% of patients and may be related to relative ischaemia of the kidney[14].

Patients with hypertension due to fibromuscular dysplasia of the renal arteries tend to be younger than those with renovascular hypertension due to atheroma. Those with atheromatous renal artery lesions in the Cooperative Study had a somewhat higher systolic blood pressure and exhibited more widespread arterial disease with more target-organ damage than those with essential hypertension. Those with fibromuscular dysplasia tended to be younger, female and without a family history of raised blood pressure. The authors of the Study concluded[12], however, that there were no truly distinctive features to differentiate essential hypertension from that due to RAS, despite the previous published reports of much smaller studies. It may be that in the future a multifactorial analysis will evolve with each factor appropriately weighted according to its significance. Even at the present, however, it is possible to select patients for further study using a multifactorial approach to clinical featutes[15], although it remains impossible to differentiate essential from renovascular hypertension on clinical grounds alone[16].

ASSESSMENT

It is important to recognize that renovascular disease is not the same as renovascular hypertension. Renovascular disease is a term which generally indicates the presence of a stenotic lesion in the renal artery or its branches; the patient may or may not be hypertensive[17]. Renovascular hypertension, on the other hand, describes a stenotic renal artery lesion in association with hypertension *that is relieved by surgical or angioplastic correction of the lesion or by removal of the affected kidney.* Renovascular hypertension, therefore, is a diagnosis that can only be confirmed retrospectively. It has already been noted that clinical features are of little help in assessing which patients have true renovascular hypertension. The present section is devoted to an analysis of the investigative techniques that might be used to increase the yield of true diagnoses and concludes with a suggested investigative plan for patients with putative renovascular hypertension. Although many assessment techniques have been suggested that might help in the diagnosis of renovascular disease and/or renovascular hypertension, only four remain in common use to any extent; the remainder have disadvantages in terms of accuracy, safety, difficulty, or cost. Of these four, isotope studies, intravenous urography (IVU), and angiography aim to detect renovascular disease, while only renal vein renin sampling is available as a potential indicator of true renovascular hypertension.

84

Isotope studies

Radioisotope renography as a screening procedure in hypertension was suggested 30 years ago[18] and the ability of the technique to detect RAS has been subjected to many clinical trials. The earlier studies depended on the fact that a poorly perfused kidney will take up, accumulate a peak concentration of, and excrete a non-resorbable solute such as ^{131}I-labelled sodium iodohippurate more slowly than will a normal contralateral kidney. A recent review[19] of nine angiographically controlled trials of such renograms involving 934 patients with RAS and 951 patients without renovascular disease has shown an overall sensitivity of 74% and a specificity of 77%.

In the last ten years, sequential renal scanning after the rapid injection of either ^{99m}Tc pentate or ^{113m}In edetic acid has been used in an attempt to improve performance, and the sensitivity and specificity of the technique may now approach 90% for the detection of significant RAS[20-22]. Although the newer isotope methods have an increased accuracy and may also provide predictive data in terms of retrieval of function after revascularization in the azotaemic patient[23], they are more than twice as expensive as rapid-sequence IVU. These tests have been used occasionally in Oxford in the assessment of renovascular disease and they offer obvious advantages for patients who are sensitive to iodine-based radiographic contrast media.

Intravenous urography

Like isotope renography, IVU does not directly demonstrate the condition of the renal artery. Both techniques rely on the physiological differences between a normally perfused and a poorly perfused kidney to allow an inference about renal vascular anatomy. RAS reduces glomerular filtration rate on the affected side, which delays the appearance of intravenously injected contrast medium in the renal calyces. The delay also allows more time for the tubular resorption of water, resulting in an increased concentration of contrast medium in the poorly perfused kidney. Along with a decrease in kidney size, these are the features seen on an IVU that allow the diagnosis of RAS to be inferred.

As a technique for assessing RAS, the IVU has been used longer than radioisotope renography[24], although results were poor before the introduction of the rapid-sequence IVU[25]. The largest single angiographically controlled study of the value of IVU in screening for renovascular disease remains the Cooperative Study of Renovascular Hypertension[26]. Rapid-sequence IVUs were reviewed in 414 patients with unilateral RAS, 244 patients with bilateral RAS and 772 patients with normal renal arteries who had essential hypertension[27-29]. The criteria of abnormality in these IVUs were disparity in renal length, disparity in calyceal appearance time or disparity in contrast medium density on late films[30]. Over all cases, a specificity of 89% and a sensitivity of 60% were achieved. If only RAS greater than 50% was considered, the rapid-sequence IVU correctly diagnosed 79% of unilateral disease and 61% of bilateral disease.

A sensitivity of less than 60% has remained a problem in some recent studies[31], while others[32] have reported a value of 78%. Controversy surrounds the technique of angiography because in many series authors have not used selective methods of contrast medium injection and oblique projections, which omission might have led to lesions being missed and IVUs being wrongly labelled as false positives as a consequence. Furthermore, not all authors have performed or interpreted the IVUs according to the Cooperative Study criteria and the degree of stenosis required for the diagnosis of RAS is variable in the literature – from 30%[33] to 50%[31]. Finally, not all reports give the relative proportion of patients with unilateral and bilateral disease. Since IVU depends on a disparity of appearance of contrast medium between the two kidneys, series with large proportions of bilateral lesions will probably achieve a lower sensitivity for IVU. A recent assessment[19] of the value of IVU has been made by reviewing all angiographically controlled series in the literature from 1962 to 1983. This identified 2040 patients with angiographically proven RAS and 2133 patients with normal angiograms who had essential hypertension. Rapid-sequence IVU achieved a sensitivity of 75% and a specificity of 86%.

There is little doubt that the rapid-sequence IVU has been in use longer and has been more extensively evaluated than any other non-invasive test for screening for renovascular disease. Although its cost-effectiveness has been challenged[34], it remains relatively inexpensive compared with competing techniques and it can be performed on an outpatient basis. While it is far from perfect, it has been routinely employed in Oxford in the assessment of putative renovascular hypertension up to the present, although modern angiographic techniques will make it obsolete. It has been under attack recently on the basis of cost as a presurgical screening measure for a disease that, some argue, might just as well be managed medically[9,35]. Others have emphasized the relatively few patients with surgically correctable hypertension and the potentially superior accuracy of newer techniques such as digital subtraction angiography[6].

Angiography

The newest method of assessment of importance in renovascular hypertension is digital subtraction angiography (DSA). This technology has made the radioisotope renogram and the IVU obsolete in many centres where DSA is now considered to be the primary method of evaluating patients with possible renovascular hypertension[36-38]. It must be appreciated, however, that DSA has been in routine use for only six years and there is, as yet, no conclusive demonstration in the literature that it has a significant advantage over the older methods. It has considerable potential as a screening method, recording radiographic exposures using image-intensification after the intravenous injection of contrast medium. Subtraction of venous images is performed by computer to visualize the abdominal aorta and the renal arteries. The procedure can be carried out quickly on an outpatient basis using either a central, e.g. superior vena cava[39], or peripheral vein for the injection of contrast medium[40]. Although DSA produces images like those of conventional angiography, it does so with much less risk or discomfort to the patient. It also requires less time and is cheaper.

Intravenous digital subtraction angiography (IVDSA) is a significant and useful advance in medical technology, but it should not be forgotten that it has several problems when compared with conventional angiographic techniques. DSA requires more patient cooperation to exclude artefacts due to motion, an unfortunately common feature of the computerized technique. Even gas moving by peristalsis through the gut has prevented proper imaging of the renal vasculature[41]. DSA also has a decreased spatial resolution that has limited its ability to identify arterial lesions in the branches of the main renal artery and in the distal aspect of the main artery itself, making it potentially unsuitable in the diagnosis of conditions like fibromuscular dysplasia[9]. In IVDSA, unlike in selective arterial injection studies, mesenteric vessels that overlap the renal arteries may make interpretation difficult without the use of additional injections of contrast medium. Such manoeuvres prolong the duration of the investigation and increase the risk of renal dysfunction induced by contrast medium or even of acute renal failure. Such complications may result from even the most straightforward of studies using iodinated contrast material. The risk of renal damage increases with dose and dehydration of the patient. Pre-study dehydration was an integral part of an IVU in the past, but this is no longer the case in most centres and the state of hydration is equivalent in patients undergoing either rapid-sequence IVU or renal DSA. However, the renal DSA requires at least 50% more iodine than an IVU and so exposes patients to a theoretically greater risk of renal damage related to contrast medium[42]. The final disadvantage of IVDSA is that it regularly produces non-diagnostic images. This is especially so in patients suffering from obesity or reduced renal or cardiac function[19].

Havey and his colleagues[19] have reviewed 13 papers, covering all the published data to 1985 on the subject of the accuracy of IVDSA in the diagnosis of RAS compared with conventional arteriograms. Four hundred and six hypertensive patients were identified who had undergone both IVDSA and conventional renal arteriography. In these studies, the sensitivity of IVDSA ranged from 75%[43] to 100%[44,45] and the specificity ranged from 76%[40] to 100%[46]. Havey calculated an overall sensitivity and specificity of 88% and 90% respectively from these studies but was careful to point out that a review of 965 instances of renal IVDSA in the literature showed 7.4% to be uninterpretable, owing to the problems with DSA discussed above[19]. If such a figure is accepted, then these sensitivity and specificity calculations are likely to over-estimate the actual performance of IVDSA.

We have so far discussed DSA only after the intravenous injection of contrast medium. While this is the important new screening test that has been hailed by some as superior to the older isotope or IVU studies, it is clear that it is far from perfect. The conventional arteriogram, obtained by retrograde catheterization of the aorta and renal vessels via percutaneous puncture of the common femoral artery, remains the 'gold standard' of assessment in renovascular disease as it does at most other sites of preoperative arterial investigation. It is worthy of note, however, that digital subtraction technology can be used to advantage in conventional intra-arterial studies. This so-called intra-arterial digital subtraction angiography (IADSA) allows the use of smaller catheters and smaller volumes of contrast medium along with a reduction in concentration of contrast medium. IADSA should probably be regarded as a safer form of conventional angiography rather than as a new technique in its own right. Arteriography by intra-arterial injection is undoubtedly the most accurate, if invasive, method of diagnosing RAS and it is likely to be required before any surgical intervention is undertaken. It is also very appropriate if percutaneous transluminal angioplasty is to be considered, since it can be performed at the same session both before and after completion of the angioplasty. In Oxford, all attempts to alleviate RAS, whether by surgery or angioplasty, have been preceded by arteriography carried out by intra-arterial contrast injection. Before 1985 this was by conventional arteriography, more recently by renal IADSA.

Conventional angiography, however, still has its advocates in terms of general screening for RAS. A recent retrospective analysis of patients with renovascular disease undergoing renal arteriography and other studies have suggested that IVU and isotope renography are sufficiently inaccurate that many patients with the condition are missed. The authors confirm the usefulness of surgery or angioplasty in the treatment of the condition and conclude that if there are no contraindications to investigation or intervention, anteriography is the only investigation that should be done to demonstrate a true stenosis[47].

Functional tests

Renovascular disease need not necessarily cause hypertension[17] and so several tests have been devised to assess the *functional* significance of an anatomical stenosis. The response to the competitive angiotensin II antagonist saralasin acetate lacks specificity and is no longer used[48,49]. Deterioration in renal function related to antihypertensive drug therapy has been reported in patients with RAS. The angiotensin-converting enzyme inhibitors captopril and enalapril in particular have been shown to cause reversible renal insufficiency in patients with bilateral renovascular disease or RAS in a solitary kidney[50] or in an allograft[51]. These observations may be explained by studies that indicate that angiotensin II mediates efferent arteriolar tone, maintaining glomerular filtration rate at low pressures of renal perfusion[52]. Blockade of the renin–angiotensin cascade with an angiotensin antagonist or converting enzyme inhibitor may abolish the autoregulation of glomerular filtration at diminished renal artery pressures[53]. It has been suggested that the long-term but not the short-term response to captopril is a useful predictor of the outcome of surgery for renovascular hypertension[54], but that prolonged exposure to captopril may permanently impair renal function[55]. It must be noted too that reversible deterioration of renal function has been associated with the lowering of blood pressure not only with converting enzyme inhibitors but also with other drugs including minoxidil and sodium nitroprusside[7]. The simple lowering of perfusion pressure in the presence of critical RAS results in a diminished glomerular filtration rate irrespective of the status of the renin–angiotensin system[56].

The measurement of supine[57] and stimulated[58] peripheral plasma renin activities has been assessed as a functional test of renovascular hypertension, but although renal ischaemia may result in raised peripheral plasma renin levels, this can be influenced by many other factors and the sensitivity of such tests is extremely poor[59]. Of all the proposed functional tests to date, only divided renal vein renin studies have been used extensively as a predictor of outcome of intervention for renovascular hypertension. This, however, is an invasive test requiring catheterization of the vena cava and renal veins. It has been available and widely used for many years, but the results achieved are conflicting[59–61]. A ratio of renin activity of greater than 1.5 between the side of the stenosis and the contralateral side has been suggested as indicating a functional stenosis, but even recent studies continue to show that such high ratios may occur in less than half the patients with RAS and in one-quarter of those with normal arteriograms[47]. In the same study, the ratio was also a poor predictor of the outcome of surgery or angioplasty because as many patients did well with a negative ratio as with a positive ratio; poor outcome in those with a positive ratio was not associated with technical failure. Other workers[62] have also shown that an improvement or cure of hypertension after intervention for RAS in patients with non-lateralizing renin ratios can be expected in 57% of cases. Some have suggested that the ratio might be especially useful in lateralizing the functional disorder in bilateral RAS, but inconclusive ratios result in over one-third of such patients[61]. In the authors' experience, renal vein renin assays have proved of value in predicting the outcome of surgical reconstruction if a high output of renin from the side of a unilateral stenosis is associated with complete suppression of renin secretion from the contralateral side. There has been a good response to reconstruction in all such instances.

All these so-called functional tests are based on the concept that renovascular hypertension is related to the renin–angiotensin system; with the exception of divided renal vein renin studies, none have stood the test of time. Even the renal vein renin assay is considered of questionable value by many and it is both invasive and expensive. The poor predictive ability of these studies may, of course, indicate that factors other than the renin–angiotensin system cause or contribute to the hypertension of RAS[63].

Planning investigation

Hypertensive individuals between the ages of 18 and 74 years probably form rather more than 10% of the total population of Western communities[64] and on grounds of safety and expense alone the assessment of such a large number of individuals using any of the techniques discussed in this section cannot be justified. Some have suggested that only moderately to severely hypertensive patients (with diastolic blood pressure 105 mmHg or greater) need be examined[65], but this is still

29% of all hypertensives[66] and would encompass nearly two million people in the U.K. If only 3% of those with elevated blood pressure have renovascular hypertension, only one individual with this disease would be identified per ten screening tests and not all of these would be suitable for surgical intervention. Some other strategy seems appropriate.

Thornbury and his colleagues[6] have suggested that patients should only be investigated if intervention by either surgery or percutaneous transluminal angioplasty is contemplated and points out that at the University of Michigan the group selected for arteriography on the basis of *operative* criteria is about three times the number actually undergoing operation, either reconstruction or nephrectomy. These figures are corroborated by Gifford[15] who has shown in a review of eight studies encompassing 3457 hypertensive patients who had arteriography that 1109 (32%) had RAS and 406 (13%) underwent surgery. The cost of any of the investigative procedures discussed in this section is not inconsequential and all the techniques are imperfect. It would be highly wasteful of resources to examine all hypertensives and some selection criteria seem necessary.

Although clinical criteria cannot be used with confidence to identify *individuals* with renovascular hypertension, certain features can be used to describe subpopulations of hypertensives which have a high probability for successful surgical correction of renovascular hypertension[67,68]. Gifford[15] has assessed the traditional clinical clues, and the following list contains the five that he considers most reliable. They are presented in descending order of likelihood of renovascular hypertension being present.

(1) Bruit in epigastrium or flank
(2) Abrupt onset or exacerbation of hypertension, with rapid progression
(3) Onset before 30 years or after 55 years of age
(4) Accelerated hypertension
(5) Arteriospastic retinal vascular changes.

The more of these features that are present, the more likely it is that RAS will be found, and using such selective criteria it has been possible to achieve 25–66% positive arteriograms for renovascular disease, although not necessarily for renovascular hypertension[15]. It should be noted in addition that patients with evidence of renal failure, including those who have reduced renal function when treated by angiotensin converting enzyme inhibitors, merit early investigation[8]. It must also be remembered that those with suspected bilateral RAS or RAS in a solitary kidney should not be treated in the long-term with such drugs, since this policy will result in permanent loss of renal function in many patients[69].

Thus, we should investigate patients not excluded from intervention for other reasons such as severe vascular disease at other sites or advanced non-vascular pathology and whose condition is not adequately controlled by antihypertensive medication along with those identified by the criteria outlined above. The aim should be to ensure that the number of patients is greater than the number of interventions for renovascular hypertension by no more than a factor of three or four.

There seems little point in careful selection of patients to ensure a correct use of resources if those selected patients undergo an inappropriately large number of tests. There can be no case for submitting putative renovascular hypertensives to isotope renography, rapid-sequence IVU, DSA and then conventional arteriography. Such a policy is expensive and distressing to the patient. Although the accuracies of isotope studies, IVU and renal IVDSA are fairly similar, only renal IVDSA results in anatomical pictures of the renal vasculature that might be of use to the surgeon. If the surgical service of the institution involved is happy to operate often with IVDSA evidence alone, as opposed to conventional arteriographic or IADSA images, then renal IVDSA must be the screening procedure of choice. On the other hand, many vascular surgeons may demand conventional arteriograms and/or IADSA imaging. If this is so, and a screening test is required, then rapid-sequence IVU may be considered because it is the cheapest. However, the accuracy of any of the screening techniques is far less than 100%, and many now believe that arteriography (conventional and/or IADSA) should be the first and definitive investigation when RAS is suspected[47]. None of the functional studies have proved to be of much use in predicting the outcome of intervention for renovascular disease. Although divided renal vein renin studies are still employed in some centres, and may be valuable in certain individual cases, they are invasive and expensive and probably cannot be justified for routine use.

SURGERY

Surgical correction of RAS can be achieved by four principal techniques. Whether transaortic renal endarterectomy, bypass grafting, arterial reimplantation or autotransplantation is employed, preoperative assessment in atheromatous cases should include careful screening for coronary artery and cerebrovascular disease, particularly in view of the reduction in perfusion pressure that may follow successful renal revascularization. If significant lesions are detected in these territories, consideration should be given to their correction before undertaking renal artery surgery. Today, in addition to formal operative intervention, percutaneous transluminal angioplasty (PTA) has also gained a significant place in the management of RAS. The remainder of this section principally concerns surgical intervention, although PTA is described briefly.

Whatever surgical technique is used, in the immediate preoperative period antihypertensive drugs should be reduced to the minimum necessary to maintain a stable blood pressure in bed, but they should not be discontinued. Severe hypertension can be controlled with nitroprusside infusion in the perioperative period. Patients with renovascular hypertension may have a depleted intravascular fluid volume, especially if diuretics have been given, and adequate fluid loading is important to prevent ischaemic tubular damage. If there is ischaemic heart disease with left ventricular dysfunction, the insertion of a Swan–Ganz catheter is advisable to allow fluid therapy to be adjusted to maintain wedge pressure and cardiac output at normal levels throughout the perioperative period. These measures should prevent myocardial ischaemia in most patients, although a few may still require nitroprusside or glyceryl trinitrate if signs of left heart strain develop during aortic clamping[70].

Most procedures carried out on the renal artery involve less than 30 minutes warm ischaemia of the kidney. If warm ischaemia is likely to exceed this time, especially if renal function prior to surgery is impaired, cold perfusion of the kidney with heparinized Ringer's lactate at 4°C may be used, with or without the addition of inosine[71,72]. However, provided that dissection is confined to the renal artery and aorta, and the kidney itself is not disturbed in its bed with its collateral supply, usually the kidney with a tight RAS will not be damaged by periods of renal artery occlusion of over 1 hour.

Transaortic renal endarterectomy

Most surgery on the renal arteries is usually carried out in Oxford transperitoneally via a long midline abdominal incision, although some prefer a transverse incision or an extraperitoneal flank approach[73]. On the left side the renal vein must be mobilized to allow access to the renal artery, and on the right the inferior vena cava must be retracted laterally. After systemic heparinization, arterial clamps are placed on both renal arteries beyond the limits of the atheroma and on the aorta below the renal vessel origins and above the origins – this last clamp is placed either at the infracoeliac suprarenal site or on the supracoeliac aorta. The aorta is then opened longitudinally at the level of the renal arteries. The endarterectomy is carried out with a blunt dissecting spatula (MacDonald's dissector), starting in the aorta and working towards and into each renal artery in turn. Endarterectomy is generally performed in the transmedial plane. As gentle traction is applied to the loosened atheromatous layer and the cleavage plane is extended into the renal artery, the renal artery is everted slightly into the aortic lumen. A more superficial plane is progressively reached and the atheromatous plaque is eventually separated, leaving the distal renal artery intima adherent to the underlying media. When clearance is complete and the distal intimal adherence is checked, the vessels are flushed with heparinized saline to remove any loose debris and the aortotomy is closed with a continuous-monofilament non-absorbable suture. A period of hypotension may result on aortic declamping and the anaesthetist should be warned in advance of this manoeuvre in order that a full fluid load can be established.

Transaortic endarterectomy has the advantage that it does not require prosthetic vascular graft material and that both renal arteries can be dealt with during one short period of aortic occlusion. It is especially suited to patients with bilateral disease. If the atheroma

95

extends beyond the proximal segment of the renal vessel, however, the distal end of the endarterectomy may be difficult to visualize and a smooth endarterectomy without a distal intimal flap may be difficult to achieve. This may lead to intimal dissection in the distal renal artery and the technique is best avoided in such cases.

Bypass grafts

Like transaortic endarterectomy, aortorenal bypass is a popular technique for renal artery reconstruction both in Oxford and in other centres. Access to the left renal artery follows similar lines, although an alternative method is to mobilize the left colon and the spleen medially. On the right side the artery is exposed after mobilizing the hepatic flexure of colon and sweeping the duodenum and head of pancreas medially off the front of the inferior vena cava. On each side the renal vein requires to be mobilized to complete the access to the artery.

The condition of the infrarenal aorta is reasonably good in many patients and a bypass graft may be attached at this site. It may be possible to attach the graft to one or other common iliac artery if the aorta is severely diseased. While the retrograde nature of the blood flow in such a graft may have theoretical haemodynamic disadvantages, this has not proved to be a significant problem in practice and infrarenal by-pass is technically easier than by-pass from a supracoeliac level. Autogenous saphenous vein harvested from the leg has produced good results as an aortorenal graft in Oxford, although some have suggested that stenosis and occlusion may occur in a small number of cases[74] and it has also been noted that autogenous vein has had limited durability when used as a by-pass to the visceral arteries[75]. Certainly, if the aorta is at all thickened, it is easier to suture a polytetrafluoroethylene or a Dacron graft to this vessel, but such grafts comprise only 8% of aortorenal grafts in the Oxford series. The high flow rates through these grafts have, however, ensured good long-term patency and the possibility of infection in the prosthetic material has been a theoretical rather than a practical consideration in this and most other series. Whatever material is chosen, after systemic heparinization and arterial clamping an end-to-side anastomosis is fashioned between graft and aorta and an end-to-end or end-to-side anastomosis between graft and renal artery, distal to the stenosis.

If the aorta below the renal arteries is heavily diseased an aortoiliac endarterectomy may be done or the diseased vessel may be replaced by a Dacron aortic graft prior to reconstructing one or both renal arteries. The graft to one or both of the renal vessels is then attached end-to-side to the aortic graft. Such combined surgery has accounted for no less than 18% of all technically successful renal artery reconstructions in Oxford and is to be preferred to the alternative of constructing an antegrade aortorenal bypass from the supracoeliac aorta[76]. The use of visceral artery branches as donor vessels for renal artery by-pass has also received renewed publicity in the recent literature. Several vessels may be suitable, such as the hepatic artery[77], splenic artery[78], gastroduodenal artery[79] and mesenteric arteries[80]. These alternative methods may appear attractive when the infrarenal aorta is too diseased to support a graft, as they seem to offer a technique of lesser magnitude than combined aortic replacement and renal by-pass. It must be noted, however, that although renal revascularization alone has been shown to carry an operative mortality rate of less than 1% in experienced hands, and simultaneous aortic and renal surgery carries an operative mortality rate of 12%[23], techniques such as splenorenal by-pass also have a combined operative mortality and failure of intervention rate of 12%[78]. In fact, when the small subgroup of very high-risk patients that can be recognized preoperatively is excluded, combined aortic and renal surgery is an acceptably safe procedure[81] and in the Oxford series no operative or perioperative death has resulted using this technique.

It would seem that the use of these alternative methods offers little real advantage at present, one exception being the use of the internal iliac artery in paediatric patients. These grafts have proved remarkably free from late dilatation and stenosis and the internal iliac artery can be regarded as the optimum graft for renal revascularization in young children[82].

Renal artery reimplantation

When the stenosis is confined to the proximal aspect of the renal artery, especially if a good length of artery is available, it may be possible to resect the stenotic portion and reimplant the distal vessel back into the aorta. This construction clearly avoids one of the two anastomoses inherent in the technical option of aortorenal bypass and it may be very suitable in a small number of selected cases. It has been used with good results in 8% of all renal artery reconstructions in Oxford and, although anatomical circumstances will not often permit such reimplantation, it is a useful and time-saving manoeuvre for the occasional case.

Autotransplantation

This interesting technique has been advocated in a number of reno-vascular pathologies, including distal branch aneurysmal or occlusive disease, previously unsuccessful repair by one or other of the techniques already discussed, and renal vessel trauma, where it has the advantage of permitting extracorporeal arterial repair[83,84]. Further suggested indications are aortic coarctation[85], aortic dissection compromising the renal arteries[86], aortic aneurysm involving the renal arteries[87], grossly diseased aorta with disease-free iliac arteries[88] and paediatric renal artery origin stenosis[89]. More controversially, renal autotransplantation has been proposed as an alternative to by-pass techniques in adult hypertensive patients with main renal artery stenosis due to atheroma or fibromuscular dysplasia[90].

Access to the kidney is gained, as usual, through a midline abdominal incision. The kidney and renal vasculature are visualized by the techniques already discussed, although in this instance the organ itself will require to be mobilized along with the proximal aspect of the ureter. After sytemic heparinization, the most proximal aspect of the renal artery and vein are tied and the artery and vein are divided to free the kidney. The ureter need not be transected in this operation unless it is intended to remove the kidney from the body to perform extracorporeal surgery on a cooled organ. Cooling is generally achieved with the ureter still intact by perfusing the organ with ice-cold Collins' solution or some similar solution routinely used in renal allotransplantation. The solution is delivered into the renal artery using a special conical catheter tip, taking care not to disrupt the vessel intima. This is continued until the perfusate draining from the divided renal vein is clear and the kidney has blanched. The solutions generally used in allotransplantation have a high potassium content of at least 80 mmol[91] and, while they are suitable for autotransplantation, some other preparations more compatible with extracellular fluid bio-chemistry should, if necessary, be employed to protect the kidney during transaortic endarterectomy or by-pass grafting when the renal vein is intact. The disadvantage of autotransplantation is that all collateral flow to the kidney is lost and warm ischaemia is cor-respondingly more harmful than in the techniques of renal revas-cularization previously discussed. Cooling is therefore essential. The kidney is transposed to the area of the ipsilateral iliac vessels, which have been previously exposed as for an allotransplant[92]. The renal vein is anastomosed end-to-side to a venotomy in the common or external iliac vein and, after excision of the stenotic area, the renal artery is anastomosed end-to-end to a mobilized internal iliac artery, although it may occasionally be spatulated and joined end-to-side to either the external or common iliac artery. The kidney after revas-cularization takes up an extraperitoneal position in the pelvis, in which its position is reversed such that its upper pole is inferior and its anterior surface posterior, with the pelvis and ureter draining upwards in the first instance. This does not appear to give rise to any problems.

The more conventional approaches to renal revascularization are preferred in most centres, although autotransplantation seems a good alternative for many of the indications discussed, especially if the vascular surgical team have additional experience in renal allo-transplantation. In Oxford, 14% of renal artery reconstructions have been carried out by autotransplantation.

General aspects and the Oxford experience

Discounting operations for RAS in renal allografts one author (P.J.M.) has carried out 60 procedures for renovascular disease. All patients in this series had hypertension, although in 29 azotemia was

present in addition. Of the 60 procedures, 51 (85%) were reconstructions, 6 were nephrectomies because reconstruction was not possible, and in 3 a laparotomy only was performed as no pressure gradient
across the stenosis or diminution in flow in the renal artery could
be demonstrated. The types of reconstruction are described in Table
3.2.

By-pass grafting was the commonest technique and was used in well
over half of the procedures. About one-quarter of the operations were
endarterectomies and the remainder were either autotransplants or
reimplantation of the renal artery. In this series, nine cases involved
combined surgery for aortic disease, either occlusive or aneurysmal.
In the earlier years three aortoiliac endarterectomies were carried out
in conjunction with aortorenal bypass, and in later years six aortic
replacements with Dacron grafts were done along with the bypass. In
the total series there were two perioperative deaths (3.9%), one from
non-reversible renal failure and one from stroke. Deaths were not
particularly associated with the magnitude of the surgical procedure –
no death resulted from any of the combined operations.

There is no preferred operative technique for RAS correction that
will suit all situations. Varying distributions of pathology and anatomy
make it necessary for the surgeon to be able and willing to undertake

TABLE 3.2 Reconstruction techniques in 51 patients operated on for
renal artery stenosis

Technique			No.	Per cent of total
By-pass grafts	aortorenal	25	29	57
	iliorenal	4		
Transaortic endarterectomy	unilateral	6	11	22
	bilateral	5		
Autotransplantation			7	14
Re-implantation of renal artery			4	8

a variety of technical procedures, often depending on what is found at the time of surgery.

Transplant renal artery stenosis

Renovascular hypertension may occur in recipients of renal allografts and although transplant RAS has been found in only 7 (1.3%) of 540 transplanted patients in Oxford, a much higher incidence has been recorded after routine angiography in a small series of patients with hypertension after renal transplantation[93]. A short stenosis at the arterial suture line is seen occasionally. This may be atheromatous and is due to reaction to suture material or a poorly constructed anastomosis. Much commoner nowadays is a stenosis that occurs distal to the suture line, the affected vessel often being surrounded by dense fibrous tissue (Figure 3.3). Although a possible explanation for this latter type of stenosis is that it results from a fibrotic response of the periadventitial tissue to the generalized allograft reaction[94], it is also possible that it is due to intimal damage as a result of rejection that in the presence of turbulence, particularly adjacent to an end-to-side anastomosis, leads to platelet and fibrin deposition and hence the beginning of a stenotic lesion. Another possibility is that unrecognized intimal damage has occurred, either due to traction during the neph-rectomy or by the cannula tip used for perfusion of the kidney after its removal. The diagnosis of renovascular hypertension from a trans-planted kidney may be suspected in the face of decreasing renal function, especially when a new bruit is heard over the kidney and severe chronic rejection has been excluded by renal biopsy. Con-ventional arteriography and/or IADSA should be undertaken, since other forms of vascular assessment are either not applicable in the transplant situation or are unreliable.

When the diagnosis is clear, if hypertension is difficult to control or if renal function is compromised, one should attempt to correct the stenosis, but it should be realized that the surgery is usually extremely difficult and should only be performed by a transplant surgeon with vascular surgical expertise. Unfortunately, experience with balloon angioplasty has not been very encouraging, presumably because of the surrounding fibrosis, but it is probably worth attempting in the

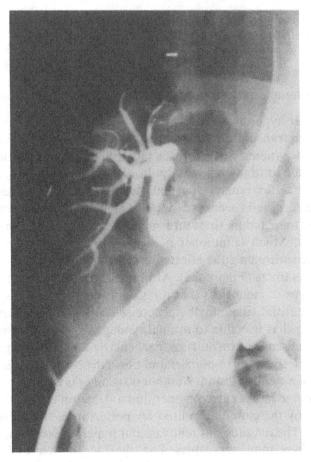

FIGURE 3.3 Post-anastomotic stenosis of the renal artery in a transplanted kidney (end-to-side anastomosis between renal artery and external iliac artery)

first instance because of the complexity of the surgery. Operative
details of this complex surgery have been described by the authors
elsewhere[95]. Eighteen (95%) out of a consecutive series of 19 such
procedures have resulted in an improvement in hypertension and 16
(89%) out of 18 patients who had poor renal function before surgery
improved also in this respect. Technical reconstruction was not possible in only one case out of 20. Thus, the results of reconstruction of

a transplant renal artery stenosis certainly suggest that this is the approach of choice provided the appropriate surgical expertise is available.

Percutaneous transluminal angioplasty

Percutaneous transluminal angioplasty (PTA) is examined in detail in Chapter 6, but it is no longer possible to discuss surgery for RAS without commenting on this interesting new technique. Soon after its introduction by Gruntzig[96] in 1978, it achieved widespread acceptance in many centres prior to the availability of follow-up data on its safety, success and durability compared with operation in similar groups of patients. Nevertheless, most authors agree that in the short term, i.e. 1 month after angioplasty, hypertension can be improved in at least 90% of patients[23]. However, when a longer follow-up is available the cure rate may fall to about 44%[97] and restenosis by 1 year has been the rule in at least one study[98].

It is doubtful whether the place of PTA in renovascular hypertension is yet clear, since long-term follow-up is not freely available for PTA-treated individuals and no controlled studies comparing surgery and PTA have yet been reported. In general, however, PTA has proved safe, allowing radiologists to proceed with balloon dilatation whenever a significant renovascular lesion is found at angiography. The logic is that PTA in such circumstances may be both diagnostic and therapeutic, but a full evaluation of this manoeuvre is not possible at present. In conclusion, there can be no doubt that balloon dilatation is a technical advance whose merits and demerits will emerge in the near future.

RESULTS

As for other diseases, the results of surgery for renovascular hypertension are dependent on patient selection. Sixty operations have been undertaken by one author (P.J.M.) in Oxford for renovascular hypertension with or without varying degrees of renal failure. In three a laparotomy only was performed as flow or pressure studies did not

103

confirm the presence of a functional stenosis. In six a nephrectomy was carried out and all six nephrectomies resulted in a cure or improvement in hypertension. In the remaining 51 operations a reconstruction of the affected renal vessel(s) was performed, with or without additional aortic surgery. Of the 51 procedures, 29 were undertaken with a primary or secondary intention to improve renal function, while 22 were solely for control of blood pressure. Four cases have been lost to follow-up or have not yet been assessed in the long term and two have died (one from stroke and one from irreversible renal failure). Of the remaining 45 (Table 3.3), a cure or significant improvement in the control of hypertension was achieved in 37 (82%). Out of the subgroup of 29 operations for which renal failure was an indication, two patients have been lost to follow-up and one has died (of irreversible renal failure). Of the remaining 26, a cure or significant improvement in renal function was achieved in 16 (62%).

These results compare well with recent reports from other centres that suggest a cure or improvement in blood pressure after surgery or angioplasty is likely in 59–95% of patients, depending on various circumstances[70,99,100]. In general, improvement in blood pressure is less likely when aortoiliac surgery is required in addition to renal artery reconstruction (59%) than when operation is carried out for isolated

TABLE 3.3 Results of reconstructive arterial surgery for renovascular hypertension ± azotaemia in 45 patients, excluding two perioperative deaths and four patients either lost to follow-up or too early for assessment from the 51 patients who underwent reconstruction (see Table 3.2)

Indication	No. of operations	No. improved[a]	
		Hypertension	Azotemia
Hypertension	19	16	—
Hypertension and azotemia	26	21	16

[a] Improved – diastolic blood pressure significantly reduced in comparison with preoperative levels such that no antihypertensive therapy was required or diastolic blood pressure was stable at less than 110 mmHg with antihypertensive therapy.

104

RAS (79%)[99]. It has also been suggested that a less favourable result is likely when the underlying pathology is atheroma (82%) than when fibromuscular dysplasia is present (95%). The outlook after surgery is also dependent on pathology. Five-year survival after correction of atheromatous lesions is 79% rising to 95% for fibromuscular dysplasia[100]. In terms of preservation of renal function, too, vascular surgery on a diseased renal artery appears worthwhile, with significant benefit for the majority of patients[7,101].

In summary, surgical reconstruction and PTA are valuable treatments for appropriately selected patients suffering from renovascular hypertension, with or without azotaemia. Because so many factors influence the management of an individual patient, it is not possible to lay down a set of rules that can be applied universally. However, in the absence of any contraindication to intervention, surgery or angioplasty should be considered whenever possible for patients with renovascular hypertension, especially in the presence of abnormal renal function, as not only may relief of hypertension be achieved, but also preservation of renal function in the long-term[100]. Our own approach is in general to attempt angioplasty in the first instance, reserving reconstructive surgery for those patients in whom angioplasty fails or in whom there is an early recurrence of the RAS following angioplasty.

References

1. Wilhelmsen, L. and Berglund, G. (1977). Prevalence of primary and secondary hypertension. *Am. Heart J.*, **94**, 543–6
2. Danielson, M. and Dammstrom, B. G. (1981). The prevalence of secondary and curable hypertension. *Acta. Med. Scand.*, **209**, 451–5
3. Rudnick, K. V., Sackett, D. L., Hirst, S. and Holmes, C. (1977). Hypertension in a family practice. *Can. Med. Assoc. J.*, **117**, 429–37
4. Gifford, R. W. (1969). Evaluation of the hypertensive patient with emphasis on detecting curable causes. *Milbank Mem. Fund. Q.*, **47**, 170–86
5. Foster, J. H., Dean, R. H., Pinkerton, J. A., Rhamy, R. K. (1973). Ten years experience with the surgical management of renovascular hypertension. *Ann. Surg.*, **177**, 755–66
6. Thornbury, J. R., Stanley, J. C. and Fryback, D. G. (1984). Optimising work-up of adult hypertensive patients for renal artery stenosis. *Radiol. Clin. N. Am.*, **22**, 333–9
7. Ying, C. Y., Tifft, C. P., Gavras, H. and Chobanian, A. V. (1984). Renal revas-

cularisation in the azotemic hypertensive patient resistant to therapy. *N. Engl. J. Med.*, **311**, 1070–5

8. Dean, R. H., Kieffer, R. W., Smith, B. M., Oates, J. A., Nadeau, J. H., Hollifield, J. W. and DuPont, W. D. (1981). Renovascular hypertension: anatomic and renal function changes during drug therapy. *Arch. Surg.*, **116**, 1408–15

9. Stanley, J. C. and Whitehouse, W. M. (1984). Occlusive and aneurysmal disease of the renal arterial circulation. *DM.*, **30**, 1–62

10. Stanley, J. C., Gewertz, B. C., Bove, E. L., Sottiurai, V. and Fry, W. J. (1975) Arterial fibroplasia. Histopathologic character and current etiologic concepts. *Arch. Surg.*, **110**, 561–6

11. Meaney, T. F. and Baghery, S. H. (1982). Radiology of renovascular hypertension. In Breslin, D. J., Swinton, N. W., Libertino, J. A. and Zinman, L; (Eds.) *Renovascular Hypertension*, pp. 78–95. (Baltimore: Williams & Williams)

12. Simon, N., Franklin, S. S., Bleifer, K. H. and Maxwell, M. H. (1972). The cooperative study of renovascular hypertension: Clinical characteristics of renovascular hypertension. *J. Am. Med. Assoc.*, **22**, 1209–18

13. Murie, J. A., Sheldon, C. D., Quin, R. O. (1984). Carotid artery bruit: association with internal carotid artery stenosis and intraluminal turbulence. *Br. J. Surg.*, **71**, 50–2

14. Shapiro, A. P., Perez-Stable, E., Scheib, E. T., Bron, K., Moutsos, S. E., Berg, G. and Misage, J. R. (1969). Renal artery stenosis and hypertension: observations on current status of therapy from a study of 115 patients. *Am. J. Med.*, **47**, 175–93

15. Gifford, R. W. (1984). Epidemiology and clinical manifestations of renovascular hypertension. In Stanley, J. C., Ernst, C. B. and Fry, W. J. (Eds.) *Renovascular Hypertension* pp. 77–104. (Philadelphia: W. B. Saunders)

16. Vaughan, E. D., Case, D. B., Pickering, T. G., Sosa, R. E., Sos, T. A. and Laragh, J. H. (1984). Clinical evaluation for renovascular hypertension and therapeutic decisions. *Urol. Clin. N. Am.*, **11**, 393–408

17. Dustan, H. P., Humphries, A. W., de Wolfe, V. G. and Page, I. H. (1964). Normal arterial pressure in patients with renal artery stenosis. *J. Am. Med. Assoc.*, **187**, 1028–9

18. Taplin, G. V., Orsell, M. M., Kade, H. and Winter, C. C. (1956). The radio-isotope renogram: An external test for individual kidney function and upper urinary tract patency. *J. Lab. Clin. Med.*, **48**, 886–901

19. Havey, R. J., Krumlovsky, F., delGreco, F. and Martin, H. G. (1985). Screening for renovascular hypertension: Is renal digital subtraction angiography the preferred noninvasive test? *J. Am. Med. Assoc.*, **254**, 388–93

20. MacAfee, J. G., Thomas, F. D. and Grossman, Z. (1977) Diagnosis of angio-tensinogenic hypertension: The complementary roles of renal scintigraphy and the saralasin infusion test. *J. Nucl. Med.*, **18**, 669–75

21. Arlart, I., Rosenthal, J., Adam, W. E., Bargon, G. and Franz, H. E. (1979). Predictive value of radionuclide methods in the diagnosis of unilateral reno-vascular hypertension. *Cardiovasc. Radiol.*, **2**, 115–25

22. Chiarini, C., Espositi, E. D., Losinno, F., Monetti, N., Pavlica, P., Santoro, A., Sturani, A., Vecchi, F., Zuccala, A. and Zucchelli, P. (1982). Renal scintigraphy versus renal vein renin activity for identifying and treatment of renovascular hypertension. *Nephron*, **32**, 8–13

23. Dean, R. H. (1986). What is new in renal revascularisation? In Greenhalgh,

R. M., Jamieson, C. W. and Nicolaides, A. M. (Eds.) *Vascular Surgery: Issues in Current Practice*, pp. 245–53. (Orlando, Florida: Grune and Stratton)

24. Poutasse, E. F. and Dustan, N. P. (1957). Arteriosclerosis and renal hypertension: Indications for aortography in hypertension patients and results of surgical treatment of obstructive lesions of renal artery. *J. Am. Med. Assoc.*, **165,** 1521–5

25. Maxwell, M. H., Gonick, H. C., Wiita, R. and Kaufman, J. J. (1964), Use of the rapid-sequence intravenous pyelogram in the diagnosis of renovascular hypertension. *N. Engl. J. Med.*, **270,** 213–20

26. Maxwell, M. H., Bleifer, K. H., Franklin, S. S. and Varady, P. D. (1972). Cooperative Study of Renovascular Hypertension: Demographic analysis of the study. *J. Am. Med. Assoc.*, **220,** 1195–204

27. Bookstein, J. J., Abrams, H. L., Buenger, R. E., Lecky, J., Franklin, S. S., Reiss, M. D., Bleifer, K. H., Klatte, E. C., Varady, P. D. and Maxwell, M. H. (1972). Radiologic aspects of renovascular hypertension: II. The role of urography in unilateral disease. *J. Am. Med. Assoc.*, **220,** 1225–30

28. Bookstein, J. J., Abrams, H. L., Buenger, R. E., Reiss, M. D., Lecky, J. W., Franklin, S. S., Bleifer, K. H., Varady, P. D. and Maxwell, M. H. (1972). Radiologic aspects of renovascular hypertension. III. Appraisal of arteriography. *J. Am. Med. Assoc.*, **221,** 368–74

29. Bookstein, J. J., Maxwell, M. H., Abrams, H. L., Buenger, R. E., Lecky, J. and Franklin, S. S. (1977). Cooperative study of radiologic aspects of renovascular hypertension: Bilateral renovascular disease. *J. Am. Med. Assoc.*, **237,** 1706–9

30. Bookstein, J. J., Abrams, H. L., Buenger, R. E., Lecky, J., Franklin, S. S., Reiss, M. D., Bleifer, K. H., Klatte, E. C. and Maxwell, M. H. (1972). Radiologic aspects of renovascular hypertension: I. Aims and methods of the radiology study group. *J. Am. Med. Assoc.*, **220,** 1218–24

31. Thornbury, J. R., Stanley, J. C., and Fryback, D. G. (1982). Hypertension Urogram: A nondiscriminatory test of renovascular hypertension. *Am. J. Radiol.*, **138,** 43–9

32. Grim, C. E. and Weinberger, M. H. (1983). Renal artery stenosis and hypertension. *Semin. Neophrol.*, 3, 62–4

33. Rufener, J., Luscher, T., Pouliadis, G., Boerlin, H. J., Meyer P., Siegenthaler, W. and Vetter, W. (1983). Practical use of intravenous pyelography in the workup of hypertensives. *Praxis*, **72,** 898–905

34. McNeil, B. J., Varady, P. D., Burrows, B. A. and Adelstein, S. J. (1975). Cost-effectiveness calculations in the diagnosis and treatment of hypertensive renovascular disease. *N. Engl. J. Med.*, **293,** 216–21

35. McNeil, B. J. and Adelstein, S. J. (1975). The value of case finding in hypertensive renovascular disease. *N. Engl. J. Med.*, **293,** 221–7

36. Hillman, B. J. (1983). Investigating the presence and significance of renovascular disease. In Hillman, B. J. (Ed.) *Imaging and Hypertension*, pp. 28–48. (Philadelphia: W. B. Saunders)

37. Gomes, A. S., Pais, S. O. and Barbaric, Z. L. (1983). Digital subtraction angiography in the evaluation of hypertension. *Am. J. Radiol.*, **140,** 179–83

38. DeSchepper, A., Parizel, P., Kersschot, E., Degryse, H., Vereycken, H. and Van Herreweghe, W. (1983). Digital subtraction angiography on screening for renovascular hypertension: A comparative study of 100 patients. *J. Belge Radiol.*, **66,** 271–9

107

39. Smith, C. W., Winfield, A. C. and Price, R. R. (1982). Evaluation of digital venous angiography for the diagnosis of renovascular hypertension. *Radiology*, **144**, 51–4

40. Buonocore, E., Meaney, T. F., Borkowski, G. P., Pavlicek, W. and Gallagher, J. (1981). Digital subtraction angiography in the abdominal aorta and renal arteries. Comparison with conventional angiography. *Radiology*, **139**, 281–6

41. Tifft, C. P. (1983). Renal digital subtraction angiography – a nephrologist's view: A sensitive but imperfect screening procedure for renovascular hypertension. *Cardiovasc. Intervent. Radiol.*, **6**, 231–3

42. Coggins, C. H. and Fang, LS-T. (1983). Acute renal failure associated with antibiotics, anaesthetic agents, and radiographic contrast agents: Radiographic contrast agents and acute renal failure. In Brenner, B. M. and Lazarus. J. M. (Eds.) *Acute Renal Failure*, pp. 301–20. (Philadelphia. W. B. Saunders)

43. Dunnick, N. R., Ford, K. K. and Moore, A. V. (1983). Digital subtraction angiography in the evaluation of renovascular hypertension. *Radiology*, **149**, 51

44. Hillman, B. J. (1982). Renovascular hypertension˙ Diagnosis of renal artery stenosis by digital video subtraction angiography. *Urol. Radiol.*, **4**, 219–22

45. Schorner, W., Kempter, H., Bauzer, D., Aviles, C., Weiss, T. and Felix, R. (1984). Venous digital subtraction angiography for diagnosis of renal artery stenosis in arterial hypertrophy: Comparison with conventional angiography. *Radiology*, **24**, 171–6

46. Clark, R. A. and Alexander, E. S. (1983). Digital subtraction angiography of the renal arteries: Prospective comparison with conventional arteriograms. *Invest. Radiol.*, **18**, 6–10

47. Carmichael, D. J., Mathias, C. J., Snell, M. E., Peart, S. (1986). Detection and investigation of renal artery stenosis. *Lancet*, **1**, 667–70

48. Carey, R. M., Vaughan, E. D., Acherley, J. A., Peach, M. J. and Ayers, C. R. (1978). The immediate pressor effect of saralasin in man. *J. Clin. Endocrinol. Metab.*, **46**, 36–43

49. Horn, M. L., Conklin, V. M. and Keenan, R. E. (1979). Angiotensin II profiling with saralasin summary of the collaborative study. *Kidney Int.*, **15**, 115s–22s

50. Hricik, D. E., Browning, P. J., Kopelman, R., Goorno, W. E., Madias, N. E. and Dzau, V. J. (1983). Captopril-induced functional renal insufficiency in patients with bilateral renal artery stenoses or renal artery stenosis in a solitary kidney. *N. Engl. J. Med.*, **308**, 373–6

51. Curtis, J. J., Luke, R. G., Whelchel, J. D., Diethelm, A. G., Jones, P. and Dustan, H. P. (1983). Inhibition of angiotensin-converting enzyme in renal transplant recipients with hypertension. *N. Engl. J. Med.*, **308**, 377–81

52. Helmchen, U., Grone, H. J. and Kirchertz, E. J. (1982). Contrasting renal effects of different antihypertensive agents in hypertensive rats with bilaterally constricted arteries. *Kidney Int.*, **12** (Supp.), s198–s205

53. Hall, J. E.. Coleman, T. G., Guyton, A. C., Balfe, J. W. and Salgado, H. C. (1979). Intrarenal role of angiotensin II and (des-asp) angiotensin II. *Am. J. Physiol.*, **236**, F252–9

54. Atkinson, A. B., Brown, J. J., Cumming, A. M., Fraser, R., Lever, A. F., Leckie, B., Morton, J. J. and Robertson, J. I. S. (1982). Captopril in renovascular hypertension: Long-term use in predicting outcome. *Br. Med. J.*, **284**, 689–93

55. Wenting, G. J., Tan-Tjiong, H. L., Derkx, F. H., De Bruyn, J. H., Man in 't Weld, A. J. and Schalekamp, M. A. (1983). Split renal function after captopril in unilateral renal artery stenosis. *Br. Med. J.*, **287**, 1413–17

56. Textor, S. C., Klimas, V., Novick, A. and Vidt, D. G. (1984). Demonstration of critical perfusion pressure for renal function in patients with bilateral renal arterial stenosis. *Kidney Int.*, **25**, 178 (abstract)

57. Nelsen, I., Nerstrom, B., Jacobsen, J. G. and Engell, H. C. (1971). The postural plasma renin response in renovascular hypertension. *Acta. Med. Scand.*, **189**, 213–20

58. Streeten, D. H. P., Anderson, G. H., Sunderlin, F. S., Mallov, J. S. and Springer, J. (1981). Identifying renin participation in hypertensive patients. In Laragh, J. H., Buhler, F. R. and Seldin, D. W. (Eds.). *Frontiers in Hypertension Research*, pp. 204–7. (New York: Springer)

59. Sellars, L., Shore, A. and Wilkinson, R. (1985). Renal vein renin studies in renovascular hypertension – do they really help? *J. Hypertension*, **3**, 177–81

60. Marks, L. S., Maxwell, M. H., Varady, P. D., Lupu, A. N. and Kaufman, J. J. (1976). Renovascular hypertension: does the renal vein renin ratio predict operative results? *J. Urol.*, **115**, 365–8

61. Pickering, T. G., Sos, T. A., Vaughan, E. D., Case, D. B., Sealley, J. E., Harshfield, G. A. and Laragh, J. H. (1984). Predictive value and changes of renin secretion in patients undergoing successful renal angioplasty. *Am. J. Med.*, **76**, 398–404

62. Marks, L. S. and Maxwell, M. H. (1975). Renal vein renin value and limitations in the prediction of operative results. *Urol. Clin. N. Am.* **2**, 311–25

63. Mathias, C. J., May, C. N., Taylor, G. M. (1984). The renin-angiotensin system and hypertension – basic and clinical aspects. In Malcolm, A. D. (Ed.) *Molecular Medicine*, pp. 178–208. (Oxford: IRL Press)

64. U.S. Department of Health, Education and Welfare: Blood Pressure of Persons 18–74 years, United States, 1971–72, Series 11, No. 150. Washington, D.C., National Health Survey, National Center for Health Statistics, April 1975. (DHEW Publications No. [HRA] 75–1632)

65. Hillman, B. J., Ovitt, T. W., Capp, M. P., Proznitz, E. H., Osborne, R. W., Goldstone, J., Zukoski, C. F. and Malone, J. M. (1982). The potential impact of digital video subtraction angiography on screening for renovascular hypertension. *Radiology*, **142**, 577–9

66. Hypertension Detection and Follow-up Program Cooperative Group. (1979). Five year findings of the hypertension detection and follow-up program. 1. Reduction in mortality of persons with high blood pressure, including mild hypertension. *J. Am. Med. Assoc.*, **242**, 2562–71

67. Stanley, J. C. and Fry, W. J. (1977). Surgical treatment of renovascular hypertension. *Ann. Surg.*, **112**, 1291–7

68. Stanley, J. C., Whitehouse, W. M., Graham, L. M., Cronenwett, J. L., Zelenock, G. B. and Lindenauer, S. M. (1982). Operative treatment of renovascular hypertension. *Br. J. Surg.*, **69** (Suppl.), s63–s66

69. Hricik, D. E., Browning, P. J., Kopelman, R., Goorno, W. E., Madias, N. E. and Dzau, V. J. (1983). Captopril-induced renal insufficiency in patients with bilateral renal artery stenosis or renal artery stenosis in a solitary kidney. *N. Engl. J. Med.*, **308**, 373–6

70. Roizen, M. F., Beaupre, P. N., Alpert, R. A., Kremer, P., Cahalan, M. K.,

Shiller, N., Sohn, Y. J., Cronnelly, R., Lurz, F. W. and Ehrenfeld, W. K. (1984). Monitoring with two-dimensional transesophageal echocardiography. Comparison of myocardial function in patients undergoing supraceliac, suprarenal-infraceliac, or infrarenal aortic occlusion. *J. Surg.*, 1 300–5

71. Brewster, D. C. (1980). Surgical management of renovascular disease. *Am. J. Radiol.*, **135,** 963–7

72. Fitzpatrick, J. M. and Wickham, J. E. (1984). Inosine in ischaemic renal surgery. In Wickham, J. E. (Ed.) *Intra-renal Surgery*, pp. 113–28. (Edinburgh: Churchill Livingstone)

73. Ricotta, J. J. and Williams, G. M. (1980). Endarterectomy of the upper abdominal aorta and visceral arteries through an extraperiotoneal approach. *Ann. Surg.*, **192,** 633–8

74. Stanley, J. C., Whitehouse, W. M., Zelenock, G. B., Graham, L. M. Cronenwett, J. L. and Lindenauer, S. M. (1985). Reoperation for complications of renal artery reconstructive surgery undertaken for treatment of renovascular hypertension. *J. Surg.*, 2 133–44

75. Wylie, E. J. (1981). In discussion of Hollier, L. H., Barnatz, P. E., Pairolero, P. C., Payne, W. S. and Osmundson, P. J. (1981). Surgical management of chronic intestinal ischaemia. *Surgery*, **90,** 940–6

76. Ekestrom, S., Bergdahl, L., Lamke, B. and Nordhus, O. (1984). The advantage of the thoraco-retroperitoneal approach for aortorenal bypass grafting. *J. Cardiovasc. Surg.*, **25,** 427–31

77. Chibaro, E. A., Libertino, J. A. and Novick, A. C. (1984). Use of hepatic circulation for revascularisation. *Ann. Surg.*, **199,** 406–11

78. Brewster, D. C. and Darling, R. C. (1979). Splenorenal arterial anastomosis for renovascular hypertension. *Ann. Surg.*, **189,** 353–8

79. Libertino, J. A. and Lagneau, P. (1983). A new method of revascularisation of the right renal artery by the gastroduodenal artery. *Surg. Gynecol. Obstet.*, **156,** 221–3

80. Khauli, R. B., Novick, A. C., Coseriu, G. V., Beven, E. and Hertzer, N. R. (1985). The superior mesenterorenal bypass in patients with infrarenal aortic occlusion. *J. Urol.*, **133,** 188–90

81. Dean, R. H., Keyser, J. E., Dupont, W. D., Nadeau, J. H. and Meacham, P. W. (1984). Aortic and renal vascular disease: factors affecting the value of combined procedures. *Ann. Surg.*, **20,** 336–44

82. Stoney, R. J., De Luccia, N., Ehrenfeld, W. K. and Wylie, E. J. (1981). Aortorenal arterial autografts. Long-term assessment. *Ann. Surg.*, **116,** 1416–22

83. Novick, A. C., Stewart, B. H. and Straffon, R. A. (1980). Extra-corporeal renal surgery and autotransplantation: indications, techniques and results. *J. Urol.*, **123,** 806–11

84. Jordan, M. L., Novick, A. C. and Cunningham, R. L. (1985). The role of renal autotransplantation in pediatric and young adult patients with renal artery disease. *J. Vasc. Surg.*, **2,** 385–92

85. Kaufman, J. J. (1973). The middle aortic syndrome: a report of a case treated by renal autotransplantation. *J. Urol.*, **109,** 711–15

86. Adib, K. and Belzer, F. O. (1978). Renal autotransplantation in dissecting aortic aneurysm with renal artery involvement. *Surgery*, **84,** 686–8

87. Purnam, C. W., Halgrimson, C. G., Stables, D. P., Pfister, R., Beart, R. W., Kootstra, G., Haberal, M., Atkins, D. and Starzl, T. E. (1975). *Ex vivo* renal

perfusion and autotransplantation in treatment of calculous disease or abdominal aortic aneurysm. *Urology*, **5**, 337–42

88. Novick, A. C., Banowsky, L. H., Stewart, B. H. and Straffon, R. A. (1977). Renal revascularisation in patients with severe atherosclerosis of the abdominal aorta or a previous operation on the abdominal aorta. *Surg. Gynecol. Obstet.*, **144**, 211–18

89. Kyriakides, G. K. and Najarian, J. S. (1979). Renovascular hypertension in childhood: successful treatment by renal autotransplantation. *Surgery*, **85**, 611–16

90. Dubernard, J. M., Martin, X., Gelet, A., Mongin, D., Canton, F. and Tabib, A. (1985). Renal autotransplantation versus bypass techniques for renovascular hypertension. *Surgery*, **97**, 529–34

91. Marshall, V. C. (1984). Renal preservation. In Morris, P. J. (Ed.) *Kidney Transplantation: Principles and Practice*, 2nd Edn., pp. 129–57. (London: Grune & Stratton)

92. Lee, H. M. (1984). Surgical techniques of renal transplantation. In Morris, P. J. (Ed.) *Kidney Transplantation: Principles and Practice*, 2nd Edn., pp. 199–218. (London: Grune & Stratton)

93. Morris, P. J., Vadav, R. V., Kincaid-Smith, P., Anderton, J., Hare, W. S., Johnson, N., Johnson, W. and Marshall, V. C. (1971). Renal artery stenosis in renal transplantation. *Med. J. Aust.*, **1**, 1255–7

94. Belzer, F. O., Glass, N. and Sollinger, H. (1984). Technical complications after renal transplantation. In Morris, P. J. (Ed.) *Kidney Transplantation: Principles and Practice* 2nd Edn., p. 407. (London: Grune & Stratton)

95. Morris, P. J. and Murie, J. A. (1986). Vascular complications after renal transplantation. In Greenhalgh, R. M., Jamieson, C. W. and Nicolaides, A. N. (Eds.) *Vascular Surgery: Issues in Current Practice*, pp. 255–65. (London: Grune & Stratton)

96. Gruntzig, A., Vetter, W., Meier, B., Kuhlmann, W., Lutolf, U. and Siegenthaler, W. (1978). Treatment of renovascular hypertension with transluminal dilatation of a renal artery stenosis. *Lancet*, **1**, 801–2

97. Tegtmeyer, C. J., Kofler, T. J. and Ayers, C. A. (1984). Renal angioplasty: Current status. *Am. J. Radiol.*, **142**, 17–21

98. Grim, C. E., Weinberger, M. H. and Yune, H. Y. (1980). Balloon dilatation as a treatment of hypertension due to renal artery stenosis: Preliminary results in 25 patients. Proceedings of the *First SCOR-Hypertension Conference, Cornell Medical Center, New York City*, March 7–8, pp. 125–9

99. Mattila, T., Harjola, P. T., Ketonen, P., Varstela, E. and Hekali, P. (1985). Isolated renal artery and combined aortic and renal artery reconstruction for renovascular hypertension. *Ann. Clin. Res.*, **17**, 19–23

100. Morin, J. E., Hutchinson, T. A. and Lisbona, R. (1986). Long-term prognosis of surgical treatment of renovascular hypertension: A fifteen-year experience. *J. Vasc. Surg.*, **3**, 545–9

101. Sicard, G. A., Etheredge, E. E., Maeser, M. N. and Anderson, C. B. (1985). Improved renal function after renal artery revascularisation. *J. Cardiovasc. Surg.*, **26**, 157–61

4

PERCUTANEOUS TRANSLUMINAL ANGIOPLASTY IN THE MANAGEMENT OF RENOVASCULAR HYPERTENSION

D. M. TILLMAN and F. G. ADAMS

INTRODUCTION

Renovascular hypertension, which probably accounts for between 1% and 2% of an unselected hypertensive population[1], not only constitutes the dual threat of severe hypertension with its complications and progressive renal insufficiency, but may also be a marker of widespread vascular disease. Until recently, the therapeutic options were limited to medical treatment with antihypertensive drugs, reconstructive surgery, or nephrectomy. Conventional drug therapy often proves inadequate for the optimal control of hypertension associated with renovascular disease, while polypharmacy and unwanted side-effects contribute to poor patient compliance. The introduction of angiotensin converting enzyme inhibitors provided a means of effectively controlling hypertension in most patients with renal artery stenosis[2,3]. Successful medical therapy, however, was associated in some instances with a decrease in renal function[4,5], and patients with bilateral renal artery stenoses or severe stenosis in a solitary functioning kidney ran the risk of developing acute oliguric renal failure[6,7].

Surgical treatment by arterial reconstruction, autotransplantation or nephrectomy is not always successful or completely free of complications. The results of the National Cooperative study[8,9] may be used to illustrate this point. Hypertension was cured in 51% of patients, improved in 15% and unchanged in 34%[8]. (Definitions of cured, improved and unchanged are given later in this chapter.) Major complications occurred in 13.1% of patients, and overall surgical mortality was 5.9%. Those with atherosclerotic renal artery stenosis had a poorer outlook, with a surgical mortality of 9.3% compared with 3.4% in patients with fibromuscular dysplasia[9]. In this and other series, nephrectomy was performed as a primary or secondary procedure in approximately 50% of patients[8,10-12]. In the light of these figures for mortality, morbidity and loss of functional renal mass, many physicians were content to rely on medical management. The introduction of percutaneous transluminal angioplasty (PTA)[13] by Gruntzig and colleagues, and the initial very encouraging results in patients with renal artery stenosis[14-18], provided a new impetus for the detection, investigation and treatment of renovascular hypertension.

In this chapter, the current status of PTA in the management of renovascular disease will be reviewed. We also report our own experience with PTA in a series of 20 patients.

DETECTION OF RENOVASCULAR HYPERTENSION

Owing to the relatively low prevalence of renovascular disease[1] in unselected hypertensive patients, routine screening is unlikely to produce a significant yield[19]. The following clinical features, however, identify subgroups of hypertensive patients in whom renovascular disease is more likely and these patients require further investigation[20].

(1) Age: young patients with moderate or severe hypertension, especially in the absence of a family history, and elderly patients with widespread vascular disease.

(2) Resistant hypertension: compliant patients whose blood-pressure control remains unsatisfactory or deteriorates despite triple drug therapy.

(3) Malignant hypertension.

(4) Unexplained renal impairment or a deterioration in renal function when blood pressure is reduced by drug therapy, especially angiotensin converting enzyme inhibitors.

(5) Abdominal or loin bruit.

(6) Hypokalaemia, unexplained by diuretic therapy or primary mineralocorticoid excess.

Intravenous urography

The rapid-sequence intravenous urogram (IVU) is still, in many centres, the investigation that provides the first objective evidence of renovascular disease. The most important diagnostic features[20] are as follows (Figure 4.1).

(1) Delay of 1 minute or more in the appearance of contrast on the affected side.

(2) Increased density of contrast, in a narrower pelvicalyceal system, due to hyperconcentration on the affected side (This is especially noticeable in later films.)

(3) Disparity in kidney size, remembering that the right kidney may normally be up to 1.5 cm shorter than the left.

(4) Scalloping of ureters due to collateral blood supply (rarely seen).

The sensitivity of IVU in detecting renal artery stenosis is only about 80%[11]. A normal study therefore, even after reviewing the films, should not deter clinicians from proceeding to arteriography if clinical suspicion remains high. The specificity of IVU is 80–90%[21,22], and therefore a significant number of patients will have an IVU with some features suggestive of renal artery stenosis, but will have a normal arteriogram.

Isotope renography

Renovascular disease can also be detected by isotope renography using radioactive iodohippurate (hippuran)[23,24]. This technique has the advantage that it is a non-invasive and relatively straightforward procedure. It relies on the fact that the renal extraction efficiency of hippuran is high, such that about 90% of the isotope is extracted on first pass through the kidney. By using a computer-linked γ-camera, measurements of total and divided effective renal plasma flow can be determined[24]. The major changes in the isotope renogram in patients with renal artery stenosis are (Figure 4.2)

(1) a shallower gradient to the uptake phase of the curve;
(2) a delay in the peak activity;
(3) slower clearance of hippuran.

The disadvantages of renography are reflected in a false negative rate of around 20–25%[11] and a false positive rate of similar proportion[23]. Renography is therefore not an ideal technique for screening patients with hypertension but it can be useful in the follow-up of patients with known renovascular disease.

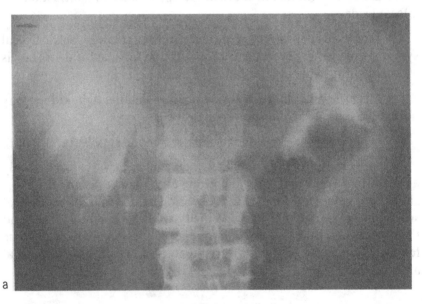

a

FIGURE 4.1(a)   IVU prior to PTA in patient no. 4 (see Table 4.6): 2-minute film showing delay of development of pyelogram on the right side. Arteriogram is shown in Figure 4.3. (b)   IVU prior to PTA in patient no. 4: late film showing increased contrast density on the right side. (c)   IVU after PTA in patient no. 4: contrast density now symmetrical

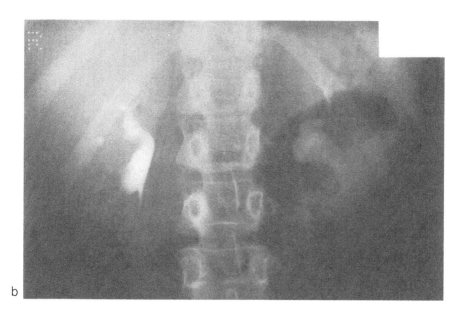

b

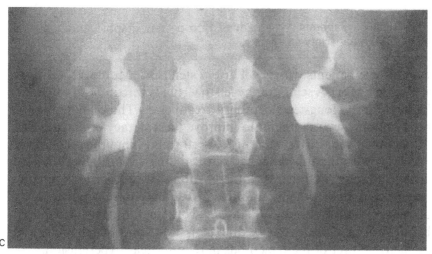

c

Renal scintigraphy with diethylenetriamine penta-acetic acid labelled with ^{99m}technetium (^{99m}Tc-DTPA) can be employed to provide measurements of total and individual glomerular filtration rates (GFR) for each kidney[25,26].

Recent studies have shown that acute captopril administration markedly reduces the extraction efficiency of hippuran on the affected

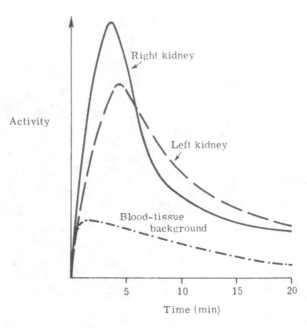

FIGURE 4.2 Schematic diagram of isotope renographic findings in a case of left renal artery stenosis

side in some patients with renal artery stenosis[27]. Moreover, GFR as measured by DTPA scintigraphy fell to virtually zero in 7 of 14 stenotic kidneys during long-term captopril treatment[27]. These findings have been exploited in an attempt to improve the accuracy of diagnosis of a 'functional' renal artery stenosis by performing hippuran renography and DTPA scintigraphy after captopril administration[28]. Early studies are encouraging, and there is an indication that captopril renography may help to predict the blood-pressure response to renal angioplasty or reconstructive surgery[28-30]. More work in this area is required before firm conclusions can be drawn on the diagnostic reliability and predictive power of these methods in renovascular hypertension.

Echo-Doppler studies

The combination of ultrasonic imaging and pulsed Doppler techniques allows qualitative and quantitative analyses of blood velocity in normal and diseased vessels, and is used clinically for the diagnosis of peripheral vascular and cerebrovascular disease[31,32]. The use of ultrasonic echo-Doppler velocimetry has been evaluated recently for the diagnosis of renal artery stenosis[33]. The presence or absence of renal artery stenosis was evaluated by an independent observer in 26 patients (52 arteries) who underwent standard or digital subtraction angiography. Compared with arteriography, the sensitivity of the Doppler method in detecting a reduction in diameter of more than 50% was 89%, while the specificity was 73%. Potential advantages of this technique are that it directly measures the haemodynamic significance of a stenosis, does not require the use of ionizing radiation or contrast medium, and therefore may be performed repeatedly to assess the progress of a renal artery lesion. It does, however, require careful and systematic examination techniques and the accuracy and reproducibility of results obtained depend on the operator. Moreover, even after repeated attempts, 11 of 68 patients (16%) had technically inadequate studies[33]; reasons for this include the presence of bowel gas, extreme obesity, significant vessel calcification and ascites.

More recently, an attempt has been made to simplify this technique by measuring the relative flow in the renal artery throughout the cardiac cycle, rather than the absolute value[34]. This obviates the necessity of measuring the angle between the Doppler beam and the vessel axis or the area of the vessel lumen. These two measurements are often difficult and may prove impossible owing to inadequate image quality. Normal and abnormal flow patterns could be differentiated by determining the ratio of peak systolic and end systolic flow volumes. This technique did not, however, distinguish between the presence of renal artery stenosis and an increased peripheral resistance due to a small kidney, nor was it capable of evaluating ostial lesions. Doppler techniques may prove useful in the follow-up of patients undergoing renal angioplasty but do not provide a reliable method of screening for renovascular disease.

Digital subtraction angiography

Digital subtraction angiography (DSA), using an intravenous injection of contrast medium[35], promised to be an effective, less invasive,

119

method of imaging the renal artery. Early studies suggested a 90% accuracy in identifying renal artery lesions[36]. Even with injection of contrast medium into the vena cava or right atrium, however, results are sometimes unsatisfactory for technical reasons[37], and poor-quality images are likely in patients with congestive cardiac failure owing to decreased cardiac output. The technique may miss ostial, branch, and parenchymal renal artery lesions[37]. Nevertheless, where available, intravenous DSA has replaced IVU as the initial screening procedure for renovascular disease, as it has in our unit. If reconstructive surgery or angioplasty is contemplated, however, complete delineation of the renal vascular anatomy, by conventional arteriography or intra-arterial DSA is preferable.

PREDICTIVE TESTS AND PATIENT SELECTION

The 'gold standard' for the diagnosis of renovascular disease is angiography. It is clear, however, that renal artery stenosis can occur in normotensive patients[38,39] and, therefore, the presence of such a lesion in hypertensive patients may be coincidental. Moreover, renovascular disease may be a consequence rather than the cause of hypertension in patients with atherosclerosis. The problem is further complicated when the natural history of Goldblatt two-kidney hypertension in experimental animals is considered[40]. In phase 1, hypertension is sustained by elevated angiotensin II levels as a consequence of excess renin production by the ischaemic kidney. In phase 2, a slow pressor mechanism is responsible for the hypertension, and plasma renin and angiotensin II levels often return towards normal. Surgery may be curative in both phases 1 and 2. In phase 3, however, other pressor mechanisms supervene, including hypertension-induced damage to the contralateral kidney. The renin-angiotensin system is less stimulated and surgery is no longer effective. It is therefore important to try to distinguish between phases 2 and 3.

An ideal predictive test in renovascular hypertension would reliably identify patients who would benefit from surgery or PTA. In practice, it should distinguish between a functionally significant stenosis and a purely anatomical lesion. It should also be able to identify significant disease in the contralateral kidney that might maintain the hyper-

120

tension after correction of the stenosis. We have previously discussed the value of the various clinical features and predictive tests in patients with renovascular hypertension treated surgically, and outlined the importance of distinguishing between diagnostic and prognostic tests[10,20].

From examination of our own and other data[10,11,20,41], there are certain clinical features that are helpful in assessing the blood-pressure response to surgery or PTA. A successful outcome is more likely in younger patients with a shorter history of hypertension and less renal impairment who smoke less and have less associated vascular disease, less cardiomegaly and less left ventricular hypertrophy.

Imaging studies

Neither IVU nor standard hippuran isotope renography are useful in predicting response to surgery or PTA[11,42], although, as previously mentioned, post-captopril renography has shown initially encouraging results and deserves further evaluation[28-30]. Arteriographic appearances of fibromuscular dysplasia, on the other hand, are likely to indicate a favourable outcome[11,14,16,18,43].

Divided renal function studies

Divided renal function studies, employing bilateral ureteric catheterization, are invasive and, although of value in establishing an ischaemic pattern, do not predict blood-pressure response[20]. This test has been abandoned in most centres, including our own. It is still advocated by some authors in specific cases; for example if renal vein renin studies are equivocal or if nephrectomy is planned for unilateral parenchymal disease[37]. In the latter case, such studies are utilized to ensure that the affected kidney contributes only minimally to overall renal function, assuring little loss of glomerular filtration following nephrectomy.

Pressure gradient

Measurement of the pressure gradient across the stenosis can provide some guide to the functional severity and the likelihood of response to surgery. Various cut-off values have been suggested, between 40 and 60 mmHg, but none has proved discriminatory.

Renal vein renin studies

Comparison of renin values in the two renal veins, popularized by Judson and Helmer[44], has been used extensively to evaluate patients with renal artery stenosis, but its value remains controversial. There is no universally accepted protocol for renal vein renin estimation. We perform the test under conditions of normal controlled sodium intake, supine posture, and, if possible, freedom from the effects of drugs[45]. Others, in an attempt to increase the diagnostic and predictive power of the test, employ various manoeuvres to stimulate renin release. These include tilting[46], sodium restriction[47], vasodilator administration[48], diuretic therapy[41] and converting enzyme inhibition[49].

Most studies of renal vein renin have relied on the ratio of renin in the two renal veins, with a cut-off point of 1.5 : 1 or 2 : 1 being taken as the upper limit of normal[10,50]. Marks and Maxwell[50], in reviewing 21 published series, have pointed out that the degree of confidence with which surgical success can be predicted depends on the ratio used: 81% confidence with a ratio of 1.5 : 1 and 95% confidence with a ratio of 1.96 : 1 or more. This parallels our own experience with surgical treatment[10,20]. However, if the renal vein renin ratio is used as the sole criterion for intervention, a significant proportion of potentially successful candidates will be denied appropriate treatment. Indeed, in Marks and Maxwell's series, 51% of 126 patients who underwent surgery despite failing to achieve a 'positive' ratio had a successful outcome.

Other authors have found renal vein ratio measurements of little value in predicting outcome of surgery or PTA. Employing a ratio of 1.5 : 1, Sellars and colleagues[11,12] found that neither basal nor stimulated renal vein renin values had any prognostic value in the surgical treatment of hypertension due to unilateral renovascular disease. The false-positive rate was 39% and the false-negative rate was 71%. Geyskes et al.[14] have reported their experience in 70 patients with renal artery stenosis selected for PTA solely on arteriographic criteria. In 37 of these patients with unilateral renal artery stenosis, in whom renal vein renin measurements were made, using a cut-off ratio of 1.5:1 there were 6/18 (33%) false positives and 13/19 (68%) false negatives. Kuhlmann and colleagues[51] also found renal vein renin measurements of little help in predicting blood pressure response to PTA in 30 patients with unilateral renal artery stenosis, although Martin et al.[17] found them helpful.

Evidence of suppression of renin release from the contralateral kidney, compared with vena caval or peripheral samples (a ratio of renal vein : inferior vena cava (IVC) of 1.0 means complete suppression), is a further guide to the blood-pressure response to surgical intervention[52]. It implies that the contralateral kidney has not been affected by the hypertension to a degree that would maintain it.

Vaughan and colleagues[53] introduced a new method of renal vein renin analysis that compares the increment of renal vein renin (V) to the arterial level (A), which is estimated from IVC samples taken from below the renal veins. This increment, expressed as $(V-A)/A$ is normally 0.24 on each side. By the Vaughan criteria, curable renovascular hypertension is defined as a value for $(V-A)/A$ of 0.48 or greater on the ischaemic side, and virtually zero on the contralateral side (usually $(V-A)/A < 0.13$). Renal vein renin concentrations were measured in a series of 46 patients[54,55]. Before angioplasty $(V-A)/A$ was 0.86 ± 0.91 on the stenosed side and 0.06 ± 0.16 on the contralateral side ($p < 0.001$). Repeat measurements 30 minutes after PTA showed that the differences had begun to diminish and at 3–6 months the secretion pattern had returned to normal in 15 of these patients. The prediction of therapeutic outcome was more reliable (sensitivity 74%, specificity 100%) using the incremental method, compared to the ratio method (sensitivity 62%, specificity 60%), but the high false-negative rate with both methods remained. Although in this study the predictive power of renal vein renin estimations was poor during long-term captopril therapy, there is some evidence that acute captopril administration may increase the sensitivity of the test[37,49,55] and may therefore help to overcome the problem of false negatives.

Assessment of patients with bilateral renal artery stenosis is more difficult. Renal vein renin estimations cannot reliably distinguish between unilateral and bilateral disease[55] and, in many patients with bilateral stenosis, tend to lateralize to the more ischaemic kidney[50,55]. This is especially true in patients in whom one renal artery is completely occluded[55]. When intervention is planned, priority should be given to correction of the lesion on the side to which renin values lateralize. Marks and Maxwell[50] concluded that, if the renal vein renin ratio clearly lateralized to the more diseased side, that side alone could be repaired with a reasonable likelihood of relieving the hypertension. It is clear, however, that many patients with significant bilateral disease will require intervention on both sides for optimal results.

Angiotensin antagonists

Angiotensin antagonists, in particular saralasin, have been used to identify 'true' renovascular hypertension and to assess surgical prognosis[56,57]. However, several authors, including ourselves, found appreciable numbers of false positive and false negative results[10,58]. The partial agonist activity of the drug and its dependence on salt and volume status often made interpretation of results difficult.

Converting enzyme inhibitors

The hypotensive response to long-term, but not acute, captopril administration, has been shown in two studies[59,60] to be a useful predictor of postoperative blood pressure in hypertensive patients with renovascular disease. The single-dose captopril test[61], which relies on an exaggerated increase in peripheral plasma renin concentration, has been used as a screening test for detecting renovascular hypertension prior to combined renal vein renin measurements and digital subtraction angiography[55]. The predictive power of this test, used alone, has not been fully evaluated.

In summary, although useful prognostic information can be gained from these tests, especially renal vein renin studies, no single test or group of tests can reliably distinguish between patients who will benefit from surgery or PTA and those who will not.

In view of the low morbidity associated with renal angioplasty and the limitations of the predictive tests outlined above, some authors suggest that, with few exceptions[14], PTA should be attempted in all patients with hypertension and renal artery stenosis[14,15]. Others agree that tests such as renal vein renin estimations are not an obligatory part of investigation prior to intervention[51]. At the other end of the spectrum, the presence of a 'functional' stenosis, demonstrated by lateralizing renal vein renin values, has been considered a prerequisite for treatment by surgery or PTA[62]. In many centres, including our own, tests to determine the functional significance of renovascular disease, including renal vein renin studies, are routinely performed. The final therapeutic decision is then made in the light of various clinical, radiological and laboratory findings, taken together.

PERCUTANEOUS TRANSLUMINAL ANGIOPLASTY

PTA was originally developed by Dotter and Judkins[63] in 1964 for treatment of peripheral atherosclerotic disease. Gruntzig and Hopff revolutionized the technique in 1974 when they developed the balloon catheter[64], and this was followed in 1978 by the first report of PTA in renovascular hypertension by Gruntzig and colleagues[13]. Since then, the technique has been used widely. The best results are obtained with a team approach involving a physician with experience in hypertension, a radiologist with expertise in vascular intervention techniques, and a vascular surgeon.

Patient preparation

Patients are usually admitted at least 48 hours prior to PTA. Antihypertensive therapy is reduced if possible, and stopped on the day of the procedure in order to reduce the risk of a precipitous fall in blood pressure which occasionally follows successful angioplasty[65]. Informed consent should include an explanation that the procedure may not cure the hypertension, and the patient should be aware that formal surgery may be necessary. In this respect, the vascular surgeon should be available at the time of angioplasty.

Procedure

PTA is carried out under local anaesthesia with fluoroscopic and angiographic control, usually via a femoral arterial approach. When severe atherosclerotic disease is present in the vessels distal to the renal arteries, or when there is pronounced downward angulation of the renal artery itself, the axillary approach greatly simplifies the procedure[66]. The renal artery is entered by a precurved selective renal catheter and a guide wire is carefully manipulated across the stenosis. The diagnostic catheter is then exchanged for the appropriate-sized renal balloon catheter (4–8 mm diameter). The balloon is dilated with dilute contrast medium at 4–6 atm within the stenotic segment, so that the profile can be observed on fluoroscopy. The pressure gradient across the stenosis is often measured before and after angioplasty and arteriography is repeated to delineate the anatomical result. Blood pressure is monitored carefully during the first 24–48 hours.

Mechanism and radiographic features of successful PTA

Sos and colleagues[5] have recently discussed the technical aspects of PTA. In atherosclerotic lesions, inflation of the balloon induces splitting of the atheroma and produces radial and longitudinal tears between the intima and media of the vessel wall[67]. The adventitia must be stretched to at least one-third more than its normal diameter to overcome its elastic recoil and achieve permanent dilatation[68].

According to Sos[5], three prerequisites for optimal dilatation are the following:

1. Balloon diameter at least 1 mm greater than the diameter of the normal portion of the artery as measured on the arteriogram. It has been suggested that such 'over dilatation' may be responsible for the lower recurrence rates observed by Sos et al.[5].

2. The pressure must be adequate to inflate the balloon to its nominal diameter within the lesion.

3. The balloon must be inflated for 60 seconds.

In the case of fibromuscular dysplasia, lesions due to the commoner medial form usually dilate easily, but those associated with intimal or adventitial fibroplasia may be more resistant[5].

PTA is more likely to be technically successful if the stenosis disappears suddenly 'with a pop' and does not reappear during deflation of the balloon. If it does reappear, redilatation is required, often with a larger balloon. The morphological appearance of the vessel on the post-dilatation arteriogram has been reported to be a better guide to long-term blood-pressure response than is the pressure gradient, or its elimination[5,16].

Adjunctive medical therapy

Arterial spasm due to guide wire or catheter manipulation may increase the risk of intimal tears and renal artery dissection. Nifedipine 10–20 mg sublingually or orally 20 minutes prior to PTA[5] or intravenous nitrates[51] have been used as preventative measures. During angioplasty, heparin 2000–5000 units is injected through the catheter to reduce the risk of thrombosis. Although various long-term therapies have been used in an attempt to prevent the occurrence of thrombosis or restenosis, there have been no controlled trials proving their efficacy. Such measures have included anticoagulation with coumarin[14,51], aspirin and dipyridamole[15,65], or aspirin alone[16]. We favour the combination of aspirin 300 mg plus dipyridamole 100 mg three times daily for at least 6 months.

Technical success – determinants

Technically successful angioplasty is usually defined as a residual stenosis of less than 50% of the vessel width on the immediate post-PTA arteriogram[16,51] or the elimination of the pressure gradient across the stenosis[17]. Overall technical success rates vary according to the series, but many authors report a remarkably high value. In the series reviewed (Table 4.1), 86% of a total of 531 patients underwent

TABLE 4.1 PTA—Technical success

Author	Total no. of patients	Success No. (%)	FMD[a] total	Success No. (%)	ATH[b] total	Success No. (%)	Reference No.
Madias et al. (1981)[c]	13	10 (77)	—	—	13	10 (77)	73
Martin et al. (1981)	31	26 (84)	8	8 (100)	15	13 (87)	17
Grim et al. (1981)	26	25 (96)	10	9 (90)	16	16 (100)	75
Mahler et al. (1982)	16	15 (94)	6	6 (100)	8	7 (87)	99
Geyskes et al. (1983)	70	68 (97)	21	21 (100)	44	42 (95)	14
Sos et al. (1983)[c]	89	53 (60)	31	27 (87)	51	19 (37)	16
Tegtmeyer et al. (1984)	109	103 (94)	27	27 (100)	75	71 (95)	77
Millan et al. (1985)[c]	16	13 (81)	13	9 (69)	—	—	74
Miller et al. (1985)	63	55 (87)	15	15 (100)	46	40 (87)	43
Kuhlmann et al. (1985)	65	60 (92)	27	25 (93)	38	35 (92)	51
Bell et al. (1987)	33	30 (91)	8	7 (88)	24	23 (92)	100
Total	531	458 (86)	166	154 (93)	330	276 (84)	

[a] FMD, fibromuscular dysplasia
[b] ATH, atherosclerotic
[c] Figures exclude partial successes

successful angioplasty. There is a uniformly high degree of success with fibromuscular lesions, 93% of 166 patients having a satisfactory technical outcome. Atheromatous lesions were amenable to PTA in 83% of cases overall, although Sos et al.[16] reported technical success in only 37% of 51 patients. The atheromatous group is extremely heterogeneous, ranging from 'arteriopathic' patients with widespread vascular disease, to those with more focal renal artery lesions, and differences in patient selection are likely to play a large part in explaining the different results.

There is general agreement that angioplasty is more likely to be successful in cases of fibromuscular disease and unilateral non-ostial atheroma. The presence of a renal artery occlusion, atheromatous stenosis at the origin of the renal artery, bilateral atheromatous stenoses, or generalized atherosclerosis, are features that significantly reduce the chances of technical success[16,18,43,69,70]. Complete renal artery occlusion, however, is not considered a contraindication to PTA in some centres, and can be dilated successfully[71].

Complications

Renal angioplasty is an invasive procedure requiring a high degree of technical skill and is inevitably associated with complications in some cases. Major complications occur in 5–10% of patients overall, and there is a mortality of about 1% that must not be overlooked when selecting patients[70,72]. An attempt has recently been made to classify complications to facilitate more objective comparison of data from different centres[72]. Minor complications are reversible within the normal recovery period after PTA. Major ones, on the other hand, either result in irreversible damage, or are reversible with surgery or an extended hospital stay. Complications are further classified as direct or indirect, according to the relationship to the procedure. The important reported complications of PTA are listed in Table 4.2.

Using the classification in Table 4.2, data from several series are presented in Table 4.3. Major complications directly related to PTA occurred in 6% of cases overall, indirect ones being less common. Overall mortality was less than 1%. As expected, complications occur more frequently in older patients with atherosclerosis than in younger patients with fibromuscular disease[70]. In the series presented in Table 4.3, where the information is available[16,43,51,73,74], the overall complication rate in a total of 246 patients with atherosclerosis was 14% compared with 4% in the 84 patients with fibromuscular disease.

Some complications, such as acute renal insufficiency induced by the contrast medium, may be avoidable with careful patient preparation. On the other hand, major complications related to renal and access artery trauma are determined more by the expertise of the operator and by patient selection, and, in many cases may be unavoidable[70]. In each case, careful observation of pulse, blood pressure, renal function (including urine output, serum creatinine and urinalysis), wound site and peripheral pulses, should be continued for 3–4 hospital days after the procedure.

TABLE 4.2   PTA – Complications

A. Direct
1. Renal artery thrombosis
2. Segmental renal infarct
3. Arterial dissection
    occlusive or non-occlusive
    renal
    access artery
4. Retroperitoneal haemorrhage
5. Arterial emoblism
    peripheral
    gastrointestinal
    microcholesterol
6. Balloon rupture
7. Access artery
    haemorrhage, thrombosis, aneurism

B. Indirect
1. Renal failure
    transient, contrast-related
    irreversible, in patients with solitary functioning
    kidney or bilateral disease
2. Hypotension
    per se
    with cerebral or myocardial ischaemia
3. Anticoagulation
    haemorrhage

TABLE 4.3 PTA—Complications

Author	No. of patients	Direct No.	Direct Major	Indirect No.	Total No.	Death No.	Reference No.
Madias et al. (1981)	13	2	2	4	6	0	73
Martin et al. (1981)	31	3	3	0	3	0	17
Mahler et al. (1986)	80	10	4	1	11	1	72
Geyskes et al. (1983)	70	8	3	0	8	1	14
Sos et al. (1983)	89	9	6 (1Nx)[a]	4	13	0	16
Tegtmeyer et al. (1984)	109	5	5	7	12[b]	1	77
Millan et al. (1985)	16	1	1	0	1	0	74
Miller et al. (1985)	63	6	5 (1Nx)[a]	1	7	0	43
Kuhlmann et al. (1985)	65	3	3	4	7	1	51
Bell et al. (1987)	33	4	1	1	5	0	100
Total	569	51 (9%)	33 (6%)	22 (4%)	73 (13%)	4 (<1%)	

[a] Nx, nephrectomy
[b] Only major complications reported

Recurrence of stenosis

The incidence of recurrent renal artery stenosis after successful dilatation is not certain since follow-up angiography is not performed routinely in all patients. Intravenous digital subtraction angiography now provides a less invasive method of imaging the renal arteries and should generate important follow-up information on the long-term anatomical results of PTA.

Reported recurrence rates vary from 5%[5] to over 70%[75.] Recurrence is more likely in atherosclerotic than in fibromuscular disease. In a series of 26 patients followed for over 1 year after PTA, angiography was repeated in 18 patients and recurrence of stenosis was shown in 1 of 6 patients with fibromuscular disease and in 12 of 12 patients with atherosclerosis[75]. According to Tegtmeyer and colleagues[18] the major determinant of a recurrent stenosis requiring redilatation is the presence on the immediate post-PTA angiogram of a residual stenosis of 30% or greater[18,77]. This probably reflects inadequate initial dilatation as follow-up studies have shown a reduced incidence of recurrent stenosis if the vessel is 'over dilated'[5,18]. If recurrent stenosis has not occurred within the first 6 months, the prospect for long-term vessel patency appears good[18,77].

Kremer Hovinga and colleagues have recently reported follow-up results on 43 patients with renal artery stenosis (33 atherosclerotic, 10 fibromuscular), 33 of whom had repeat angiography 4–45 (mean 19 ± 12) months after PTA[76]. Recurrent stenosis was found in 42% of patients with atherosclerosis and 22% of those with fibromuscular disease. In contrast to earlier reports by Tegtmeyer *et al.*[18,77], neither the presence of generalized atherosclerosis, nor the extent to which the stenosis was dilated, appeared to influence the occurrence of recurrent atheromatous disease[78]. Nevertheless, the consensus view is that the technical adequacy of the dilatation is a major determinant of the risk of recurrent stenosis.

Blood pressure response

The blood-pressure response to PTA depends on a number of factors including patient selection, type of lesion, experience of the angiographer, assessment criteria and length of follow-up. It must be pointed out that the blood-pressure data in many of the studies are not as strictly controlled as in other studies of hypertension. Follow-up blood pressures are often recorded at the outpatient clinic by different doctors using standard mercury sphygmomanometers, which do not eliminate observer bias. Also, it is difficult to evaluate patients who continue to require antihypertensive therapy after dilatation. In many cases, different drugs are used before and after the procedure and this makes it difficult to assess objectively the role of PTA in any observed change in blood pressure.

Arterial pressure usually falls immediately after dilatation, but the initial response does not necessarily predict long-term outcome. It is important to monitor patients carefully after discharge, as anti-hypertensive treatment has often been stopped, and severe hypertension may supervene. According to Sos and colleagues[16], the appearance of the renal artery on immediate post-PTA angiography is one of the most important determinants of therapeutic success. In their experience, there is unlikely to be any improvement in blood pressure if a stenosis of 50% or more remains. It is also clear that patients with fibromuscular dysplasia fare better than those with atherosclerotic disease[14,16,62].

Comparison observations of blood-pressure response between different centres has been hampered by the use of different criteria in assessment. Most groups, but by no means all, use the criteria outlined by the National Cooperative Study of Renovascular Hypertension[79] as follows:

(1) Cured: diastolic blood pressure 90 mmHg or less on no anti-hypertensive treatment;
(2) Improved: a decrease in diastolic blood pressure of at least 15% but medication still required;
(3) Unchanged: failure to achieve the above criteria.

The therapeutic outcome in a total of 165 patients with fibromuscular dysplasia is presented in Table 4.4. In each series the mean follow-up was over 1 year and some patients were followed for up to 5 years[62]. In fibromuscular disease, angioplasty cured or improved 87% of all patients and 92% of those undergoing successful dilatation. Hypertension was cured in over 50% of patients. The figures for

TABLE 4.4 PTA – Blood-pressure response[a], fibromuscular disease

Author	No. of patients	Successful dilatation	Cured No. (%)	Improved No. (%)	Unchanged[b] No. (%)	Mean follow-up (months)	Reference No.
Martin et al. (1981)	8	8	5 (62)	1 (13)	2 (25)	13	17
Mahler et al. (1982)	6	6	5 (83)	0 (0)	1 (17)	19	99
Geyskes et al. (1983)	21	21	10 (48)	10 (48)	1 (4)	range 12–48	14
Sos et al. (1983)	31	27	16 (52)	9 (29)	6 (19)	16	16
Tegtmeyer et al. (1984)	27	27	10 (37)	17 (63)	0 (0)	24	77
Millan et al. (1985)	13	12	8 (62)	3 (23)	2 (15)	37	74
Kuhlmann et al. (1985)	25	22	11 (44)	7 (28)	7 (28)	14	51
Grim et al. (1986)	26	26	15 (57)	9 (35)	2 (8)	26	62
Bell et al. (1987)	8	7	5 (62)	2 (25)	1 (13)	19	100
Total	165	156 (95%)	85 (52)	58 (35)	22 (13)		

[a] Criteria for cured, improved, unchanged not always the same
[b] Includes technical failures

TABLE 4.5 PTA – Blood-pressure response[a], atherosclerosis

Author	No. of patients	Successful dilatation	Cured No. (%)	Improved No. (%)	Unchanged[b] No. (%)	Mean follow-up (months)	Reference No.
Madias et al. (1981)	13	10	3 (23)	10 (77)	0 (0)	7	73
Martin et al. (1981)	15	13	2 (13)	4 (27)	9 (60)	13	17
Mahler et al. (1982)	8	7	1 (13)	5 (62)	2 (25)	24	99
Geyskes et al. (1983)	44	42	4 (9)	19 (43)	21 (48)	range 12–48	14
Sos et al. (1983)	51	19	7 (14)	10 (19)	34 (67)	16	16
Tegtmeyer et al. (1984)	65	61	15 (23)	46 (71)	4 (6)	24	77
Kuhlmann et al. (1985)	34	31	9 (27)	15 (44)	10 (29)	27	51
Grim et al. (1986)	27	27	1 (4)	7 (26)	19 (70)	35	62
Bell et al. (1987)	24	22	3 (13)	13 (54)	8 (33)	18	100
Total	281	232 (83%)	45 (16)	129 (46)	107 (38)		

[a] Criteria for cured, improved, unchanged not always the same
[b] Includes technical failures

atherosclerotic renovascular disease are shown in Table 4.5. Only 16% of all patients were cured of hypertension. Overall, 62% of patients were thought to have benefited from the procedure (cured or improved) and this figure increased to 75% for those undergoing technically successful PTA, emphasizing the importance of achieving a good initial angioplasty result.

Renal function

Renal revascularization may also be indicated to preserve or improve renal function. This is especially important in patients with athero-sclerotic disease, which is progressive in 36–63% of patients[80,81]. Recent evidence suggests that progression occurs at a constant rate and that total arterial occlusion is more likely in patients with a greater than 75% stenosis at the outset[82]. Timely intervention in these patients may help to preserve relatively normal renal function. In addition, renal failure may be avoided, or indeed, kidney function may be improved in patients with bilateral disease, or a stenosis to a solitary functioning kidney. In this respect, it is important that renovascular disease is considered as a cause of unexplained renal failure, since revascularization may obviate the need for dialysis. The common form of medial fibromuscular dysplasia, although often bilateral, rarely progresses to total occlusion and prevention of renal failure is, therefore, not an indication for intervention[82].

Experience with PTA in the prevention of renal failure is limited. Kuhlmann and colleagues[51] have recently reviewed the effects of PTA on renal function in 42 patients followed for a mean period of 19 months. Overall renal function improved significantly in patients with fibromuscular disease and also in those with atherosclerosis. Sos *et al.*[16] have also reported an average 12% increase in kidney size at a mean follow-up of 22 months after PTA in 15 patients, suggesting that angioplasty may indeed help to preserve functional renal mass, in addition to reducing blood pressure.

The presence of renal impairment plays a major role in the decision to intervene in some patients with bilateral renovascular disease or with stenosis of the artery to a solitary kidney. These patients are often elderly, and have widespread atheromatous disease that affects

136

cerebral, coronary and peripheral circulation. Surgical morbidity and mortality is high in this group of patients and PTA was welcomed as a means of preserving renal function without running the risks of formal surgery. In a series of 34 patients with renal impairment undergoing PTA, in 11 of whom the primary reason for treatment was renal insufficiency, 18 had 'improved renal function' after the procedure[77]. More recently, a dissociation between blood pressure and renal function responses to PTA has been demonstrated[76]. Renal function remained improved up to two years after angioplasty in half of a group of eight patients with complicated renovascular disease, despite the fact that blood pressure was not changed by the procedure. Six of the patients, including five with a contralateral renal artery occlusion, had bilateral renovascular disease with successful dilatation on one side only.

Pickering and colleagues[83] have recently reported results of PTA in 55 patients with atherosclerotic renovascular hypertension and progressively worsening renal function. Technical success was achieved in 45 cases and in 26 patients (47%) there was a decrease in serum creatinine concentration that was maintained over 2–3 years' follow-up. Blood-pressure control also improved. In 5 patients (9%) there was an acute but sustained deterioration in renal function, although there were no deaths directly related to the procedure. The authors concluded that the benefit–risk ratio of 47:9 justified the use of PTA in this high-risk group.

On the other hand, Weinberger and associates[84] have reported the outcome of PTA 1–72 months after the procedure in 14 patients with renovascular hypertension complicated by renal impairment and/or a non-functioning kidney. Only 4 patients (29%) showed an improvement in blood pressure and renal function. In the first month after angioplasty, 5 patients required dialysis because of deterioration in renal function, 4 of whom subsequently died. The authors point out that these results are worse than those obtained with formal surgery and propose that PTA should be used in this group of patients only if surgery is not an option.

PTA IN TRANSPLANT RENAL ARTERY STENOSIS

Transplant renal artery stenosis has been reported in between 1% and 25% of patients[85,86] and the overall incidence has been estimated at about 10%[86]. This can cause hypertension and threaten renal function. Hypertension is common in renal transplant recipients, but features that suggest a renal artery lesion include severe drug resistant hypertension, hypertension of sudden onset, and the appearance of a bruit and hypertension late after transplantation. A bruit has been reported in 78–88% of patients with transplant renal artery stenosis but can occur with at least 20% of renal allografts in normotensive patients[86,87].

The diagnosis of transplant renal artery stenosis is usually made by conventional angiography and it is especially important in these patients to maintain adequate hydration and to keep contrast medium to a minimum to reduce the risk of nephrotoxicity. Intravenous digital subtraction angiography has been used for the identification of transplant artery stenosis[88], but the limitations mentioned earlier in this chapter make standard angiography, or intra-arterial DSA, advisable prior to any intervention.

There are essentially two types of stenosis[89,90]. The first is a short stenosis in an end-to-end anastomosis to the hypogastric artery. The second lesion is a smooth tubular stenosis that occurs in an end-to-side anastomosis to the external iliac artery. The causes of the stenosis include donor-recipient suture narrowing, vascular fibrosis caused by ischaemia or immunological injury, vessel trauma or progressive atherosclerosis in recipient vessels[70,86].

Surgical revision can be a formidable task in these immuno-compromised patients and can risk loss of renal function. Percutaneous renal transplant angioplasty is an attractive alternative and is usually possible via a femoral approach from either the ipsilateral or contralateral side, depending on the position of the anastomosis[91]. The lesions in transplant recipients are often particularly firm and difficult to dilate, but even a small increase in the diameter of the lumen can significantly improve renal function and control hypertension[92].

Mollenkopf and colleagues[93] reported technically successful PTA in 13 of 17 patients with transplant artery stenosis. In 12 of these patients blood pressure was significantly improved (mean $184 \pm 5/118 \pm 9$ to $133 \pm 13/89 \pm 11$, $p < 0.001$) and in 10 patients blood pressure remained improved on follow-up at 8–35 months (mean 21 months). Mean serum creatinine concentration improved after PTA in 4 patients who had abnormal pretreatment values.

Dafoe and colleagues[94] reported technically successful PTA in 15 of 16 patients with transplant renal artery stenosis. In 9 of these patients, both mean systolic (194 ± 22 to 134 ± 18 mmHg, $p < 0.001$) and mean diastolic (116 ± 13 to 86 ± 10 mmHg, $p < 0.001$) blood pressures were significantly reduced, and mean serum creatinine concentration was reduced in 7 patients. Complications in these two series were few, with four episodes of transient acute tubular necrosis and three haematomas.

Flechner[70] reported the experience with PTA in the four cases of significant allograft renal artery stenosis occurring in the last 350 transplants at the University of Texas Medical School at Houston. The procedure was technically successful in only one patient and in this case a femoral artery laceration required open surgical repair. Another patient developed a dissection and partial renal artery thrombosis and underwent immediate surgical resection and reanastomosis. Other authors have reported complications that include acute tubular necrosis, dissections, thrombosis, and graft loss[95–97].

In summary, PTA can be a useful and effective alternative to surgical repair of transplant renal artery stenosis and is the first-line treatment in some centres[86], although other workers are more cautious[70]. If angioplasty is unsuccessful, there is in most cases still the option of surgical repair, if medical management is deemed unsatisfactory.

PTA – EXPERIENCE OF THE MRC BLOOD PRESSURE UNIT

Patients and methods

Between March 1983 and August 1986, 20 hypertensive patients with renovascular disease who were investigated in our unit underwent renal angioplasty as the primary procedure. The initial diagnosis was made by conventional ($n = 17$) or digital subtraction ($n = 3$) angiography. The diagnosis of an atheromatous or fibromuscular lesion was based on the arteriographic appearance. The degree of stenosis, its length, and the distance from the renal artery origin were also

TABLE 4.6 PTA – Experience of the MRC Blood Pressure Unit, demographic data

Patient No.	Age (years)	Sex	Type	Diagnosis	Arterial disease	Basal BP (mmHg)	Basal serum creatinine (μmol/l)
1	45	M	FMD	L. main	IHD[a]	180/110[b] (200/128)	109
2	40	M	FMD	R. upper	—	140/92[b] (198/112)	99
3	38	M	FMD	R. lower	—	136/84[b] (140/102)	72
4	34	F	FMD	R. main	—	170/102[b] (166/98)	83
5	32	F	FMD	R. main	—	144/96[b] (196/116)	66
6	49	F	FMD	R. main / L. main	CVA[a]	182/114	91
7	44	M	FMD	L. main	—	198/120	103
8	61	M	Ath	R. main	CVA, IHD, PVD[a]	186/112[b] (170/110)	160
9	58	M	Ath	L. main	IHD[a]	240/140	88
10	58	F	Ath	R. main	IHD[a]	184/86[b] (216/106)	85
11	26	M	?	L. main / R. main	—	144/84[b]	103
12	45	F	Ath	R. occ[a] / L. lower	IHD[a]	158/80[b] (190/124)	109
13	57	F	Ath	R. main / L. main	IHD, PVD[a]	222/106	172
14	57	M	Ath	R. main / L. main	IHD[a] (vein graft) PVD[a]	216/114	258
15	49	M	Ath	L. main / R. upper	TCI, PVD[a]	216/120	133
16	65	F	Ath	R. occ[a] / L. main	IHD[a]	222/78	222
17	68	F	Ath	L. occ[a] / R. main	IHD, PVD[a]	262/110	163
18	59	M	Ath	L. occ[a] / R. main	PVD[a]	170/92[b] (216/134)	380
19	57	F	Ath	R. Nx[a]	—	160/94[b] (182/102)	352
20	62	M	Ath	R. occ[a] / L. main	CVA, IHD[a]	196/110	538

[a] OCC, occlusion; CVA, cerebrovascular accident; TCI, transient cerebral ischaemia; Nx, nephrectomy; IHD, ischaemic heart disease; PVD, peripheral vascular disease
[b] On ACE inhibitor

assessed from the arteriogram. The angle at which the renal artery emerged from the aorta, which the balloon catheter had to negotiate, was measured and was corrected for an axillary approach in two cases.

During the initial diagnostic work-up [123I]hippuran renography[24] was performed and this was repeated, where relevant, after PTA. Renal vein sampling[98] was also performed prior to angioplasty ($n = 16$) and plasma active renin concentration (normal range 10–50 μU/ml) was measured as previously described[98].

The baseline demographic data are shown in Table 4.6. The study comprised 11 males and 9 females with a mean age of 50 ± 12 (S.D.) years. Seven patients had fibromuscular dysplasia, 12 had atheromatous lesions, and in one case the aetiology was uncertain. Eleven patients had bilateral disease, 9 of whom had atherosclerosis; a contralateral renal artery occlusion was present in 5 of these 9 patients and one had previously undergone a nephrectomy for renovascular disease. The presence of renal impairment played a significant role in the decision to recommend angioplasty in eight cases (patients 13–20), while renal failure, or a recent deterioration in renal function, was the prime reason for intervention in five cases (patients 16–20). Several of the patients with atheromatous stenoses had concomitant coronary and/or cerebrovascular disease and were considered high-risk surgical candidates, while patients 17 and 20 were deemed too ill for formal surgery.

Basal blood-pressure values are means of the last two outpatient readings taken prior to PTA except in patient 17, for whom inpatient blood pressures were used. Serial blood-pressure readings measured at the outpatient clinic were used for follow-up. For patients whose treatment prior to angioplasty included an angiotensin converting enzyme inhibitor, the mean value of the last two outpatient blood pressures measured on conventional therapy are also shown. The criteria used for evaluation of the blood pressure response to treatment are those of the National Cooperative Study of renovascular hypertension outlined earlier in this chapter.

Seventeen patients underwent PTA in the Western Infirmary, Glasgow, and the remaining three were treated at the Royal Infirmary, Edinburgh. In each case, angioplasty was only attempted on one side, even in patients with bilateral disease. Angioplasty was not attempted on any occluded renal arteries. Our patients were usually admitted at least two days prior to PTA and antihypertensive therapy stopped on the morning of the procedure, to minimize the risk of profound hypotension. PTA was performed under local anaesthesia via the femoral artery in 18 patients and via the axillary artery (after a failed attempt via the femoral artery) in the other two cases. Systemic heparinization, 5000 units, was used during PTA and thereafter the patients were prescribed aspirin 300 mg daily and dipyridamole 100 mg three times daily ($n = 17$) to be continued for 6 months. Two patients received dipyridamole alone, because of allergy to or intolerance of aspirin.

Technical outcome

Of the 20 attempted renal angioplasties 11 (55%) were technically successful (Figure 4.3). In 5 of the 9 technical failures it proved impossible to pass the balloon catheter across the stenosis. Table 4.7 summarizes the clinical features of patients undergoing technically successful PTA in comparison with those in whom the procedure failed. In general, technical success was more likely in patients with fibromuscular disease and unilateral non-ostial stenosis and when the indication for dilatation was hypertension rather than renal impairment. In patients with fibromuscular dysplasia, 5 of 7 angioplasties (71%) were technically successful, compared with 5 of 12 (42%) of those with atherosclerosis. The technical success rate for unilateral non-ostial stenosis, irrespective of aetiology, was 7 out of 8 (88%), and that for bilateral atheromatous and/or ostial stenosis was 2 out of 10 (20%).

Technical failure was associated with a trend towards longer, more severe stenosis, but there was little difference between the two groups in the size of the affected kidney or in the angle subtended by the renal artery and the aorta. Coincidental arterial disease, cigarette-smoking, and an abnormal ECG were all common in both groups of patients but were more prevalent in the patients experiencing technical failure.

A striking feature was seen in the subset of patients in whom it was impossible to pass the balloon catheter (Table 4.7). All five had bilateral atheromatous stenoses with an ostial lesion on the side of

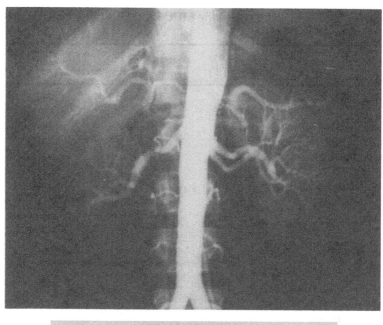

FIGURE 4.3   Renal angiographic appearance (*a*) before and (*b*) immediately after PTA in patient no. 4

143

TABLE 4.7   PTA – Experience of the MRC Blood Pressure Unit, technical success versus failure

	Success (n=11)	Failure (n=9)	FTPB[a] (n=5)
Age (years)	49 ± 13[c]	52 ± 11[c]	58 ± 7[c]
Sex	7M : 4F	4M : 5F	2M : 3F
Atheromatous (%)	5 (45)	7 (78)	5 (100)
Fibromuscular (%)	5 (45)	2 (22)	0 (0)
Bilateral (%)	4 (36)	7 (78)	5 (100)
Unilateral (%)	7 (64)	2 (22)	0 (0)
Lesion at origin (%)	2 (18)	7 (78)	5 (100)
Angle (degrees)	78 ± 24[c]	69 ± 17[c]	64 ± 14[c]
Severity[b]	2 Mild, 8 Mod	4 Severe, 5 Mod	3 Severe, 2 Mod
Length of stenosis (cm)			
<1	5	2	1
1–2	5	5	3
>2	0	2	1
Kidney size (cm)	12.2 ± 1.7[c]	12.1 ± 1.9[c]	12.3 ± 1.3[c]
Serum creatinine concentration (μmol/l)	136 ± 92[c]	213 ± 150[c]	223 ± 83[c]
Other arterial disease (%)	7 (64)	6 (67)	4 (80)
Current smoker (%)	6 (55)	7 (78)	4 (80)
Abnormal ECG (%)	6 (55)	7 (78)	4 (80)
Renal indication (%)	2 (18)	6 (67)	5 (100)

[a] FTPB, failure to pass balloon catheter
[b] Mild <50% stenosis; Mod 50–80% stenosis; Severe >80% stenosis
[c] Values are mean ± SD

attempted dilatation. Renal impairment was a major factor in the decision to intervene in each case, and in four cases there was evidence of widespread vascular disease.

Complications

Complications of PTA occurred in six patients (Table 4.8). Patient no. 2 had an unsuccessful attempt at dilating an upper polar artery. Thereafter he developed loin pain, haematuria, and a drop in haemoglobin of 4 g/dl. Subsequent digital subtraction angiography confirmed

TABLE 4.8 PTA – Experience of the MRC Blood Pressure Unit, complications

Patient No.	Technical outcome	Complication(s)	Outcome
2	Failure	Polar infarction	BP controlled on ACE inhibitor
5	Failure	R. renal a. occlusion R. femoral a. occlusion	Nephrectomy
8	Success	Segmental infarct	Asymptomatic, benefited from procedure
13	FTPB[a]	R. renal a. occlusion	Emergency by-pass graft
17	FTPB[a]	R. femoral a. occlusion	Died 8 days later
19	FTPB[a]	Transient deterioration in renal function	By-pass graft at 1 week

[a] FTPB, failure to pass balloon catheter

complete occlusion of the upper polar artery and he remains normotensive on enalapril on follow-up at 42 months. Patient no. 5, a young woman with a very long stenosis due to medial fibromuscular dysplasia (Figure 4.4(a)) experienced both renal and femoral arterial occlusion (Figure 4.4(b), (c)) during attempted PTA. Reconstructive surgery was not possible and she therefore underwent nephrectomy and femoral embolectomy. Two years later she remains normotensive on verapamil alone.

Patient no. 8 had a successful dilatation of a main renal artery stenosis but sustained a segmental infarct, presumably of embolic origin. Despite this, his blood pressure remains improved, albeit with increased drug therapy, 19 months after the procedure. In patient no. 13 it proved impossible to pass the balloon catheter and a main renal artery occlusion occurred during catheter manipulation, necessitating emergency by-pass surgery.

Patient no. 17 had widespread atherosclerosis, a left renal artery occlusion with no collateral supply, and a tight right renal artery stenosis (Figure 4.5(a)). Neither her severe hypertension nor her left ventricular failure could be controlled without a deterioration in renal

145

function. PTA was undertaken in an attempt to improve renal function but, although a guide wire could be passed through the stenosis, the balloon could not. She sustained a femoral artery occlusion during the procedure and thereafter her condition deteriorated and she died 8 days later. Postmortem examination confirmed the extensive atheromatous disease (Figure 4.5(*b*)), and the femoral artery occlusion, but the stenosed right renal artery was still patent.

Patient no. 19 experienced deterioration in renal function without renal artery occlusion following an unsuccessful attempt at dilatation (serum creatinine increased from 393 to 663 μmol/l), although this was already improving (serum creatinine 483 μmol/l) at the time of bypass grafting 1 week later.

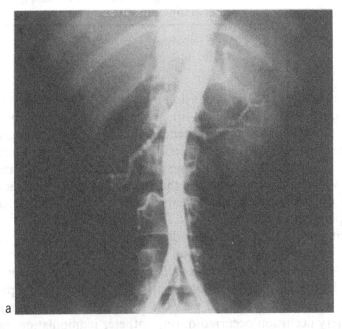

FIGURE 4.4 (*a*) Predilatation arteriography in patient no. 5 showing the long right renal artery stenosis due to fibromuscular dysplasia. (*b,c*) Immediate post-dilatation arteriogram in patient no. 5 showing the right renal artery occlusion (*b*) and the right femoral artery occlusion (*c*). Note that the lower limb arteries show evidence of fibromuscular disease bilaterally

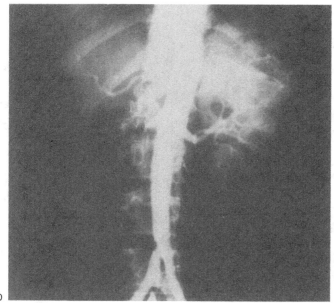

b

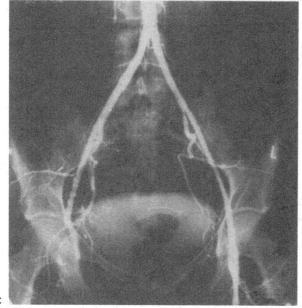

c

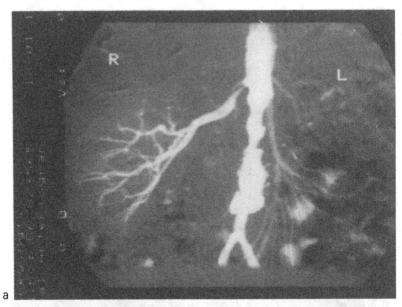

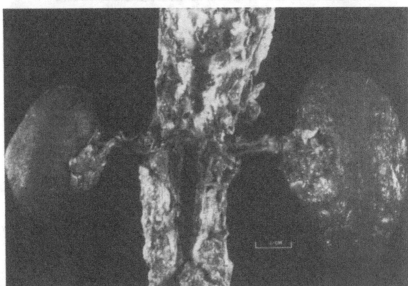

FIGURE 4.5 (*a*) Predilatation arteriogram in patient no. 17 showing severe atheromatous disease in the aorta, a left renal artery occlusion and a tight right renal artery stenosis. (*b*) Postmortem appearance of aorta, renal arteries and kidneys in patient no. 17 viewed from behind

148

Blood-pressure and renal-function response

Of the initial 20 patients in whom angioplasty was attempted 3 (15%) were cured, 5 (25%) had improved blood pressure control and blood pressure remained unchanged in the remaining 12 (60%). Table 4.9 shows details of the 11 patients in whom angioplasty was technically successful, followed for a period of 7–34 months (mean 17 ± 10 S.D.). The figures for patients undergoing technically successful PTA are, therefore, 27% cured, 46% improved and 27% unchanged.

In patient no. 16, however, who had bilateral atheromatous disease, the major indication for angioplasty was renal failure. Renal function significantly improved following the procedure, and remained so 34 months later. Patient no. 18, who also had bilateral atheromatous disease, experienced an acute deterioration in renal function during treatment with captopril prior to PTA. Renal function markedly improved after angioplasty (Table 4.9), but, as the angiotensin converting enzyme inhibitor had been stopped, it was not possible to assess accurately the effect of PTA in this respect.

In 8 of the remaining 9 patients, renal function was little altered by successful angioplasty. The mean $\pm$ S.D. serum creatinine concentration (μmol/l) in this group was 99 ± 26 prior to PTA and 96 ± 26 after the procedure.

CONCLUSION

Percutaneous transluminal angioplasty offers an effective treatment for patients with renovascular hypertension and is associated with low morbidity and mortality. Eighty-seven per cent of all patients with fibromuscular dysplasia in whom PTA is attempted benefit from the procedure, which compares favourably with surgical results. In patients with atherosclerosis, 62% of *all* patients gain benefit, and this figure increases to 75% in those patients in whom angioplasty is technically successful.

Many would regard PTA as the treatment of choice for patients with renovascular hypertension due to fibromuscular dysplasia or non-ostial focal atheromatous stenosis. However, no randomized controlled trials have been reported comparing PTA with either surgical or medical therapy.

149

TABLE 4.9 Technically successful PTA – blood-pressure and renal-function response

Patient No.	Blood pressure		Drugs		Classification	Serum creatinine (µmol/l)		Follow-up (months)
	Pre	Post	Pre	Post		Pre	Post	
1	180/110	150/92	Enalapril, sorbitrate	Nil	Improved	109	85	8
3	136/84 140/102ᵃ	124/88	Enalapril, atenolol	Nil	Cured	72	89	33
4	170/102	116/78	Enalapril	Atenolol	Improved	83	68	23
6	182/114	154/100	Tenoretic, nifedipine	Thiazide	Improved	91	82	14
7	198/120	114/82	Propranolol, hydralazine	Nil	Cured	103	115	9
8	186/112	176/88	Captopril, prazosin, frusemide	Captopril, atenolol, nifedipine, diumide-K	Unchanged	160	152	19
9	240/140	196/104	Atenolol, frusemide, minoxidil	Tenoretic, nifedipine, minoxidil	Improved	88	95	12
10	216/106	164/82	Atenolol, thiazide, hydralazine	Nifedipine	Improved	85	84	7
11	144/84	142/90	Enalapril	Nil	Cured	103	—	14
16	222/78	160/72	Metoprolol, hydralazine, frusemide	Metoprolol, prazosin, frusemide	Unchanged	222	171	34
18	170/92	186/94	Captopril, atenolol, hydralazine, frusemide	Atenolol, hydralazine, frusemide	Unchanged	380	115	12

ᵃBlood pressure on atenolol alone

The procedure fails most often in patients with ostial lesions, renal artery occlusion and long atheromatous stenoses. In this group of patients, many of whom are elderly, with widespread atherosclerosis and renal insufficiency, surgical results are also poor, and morbidity and mortality high. The benefit–risk ratio of PTA in these patients must therefore be considered carefully. Some patients in this group may be more appropriately managed with medical treatment, especially if a first attempt at PTA ends in failure. Further intervention, with surgery or angioplasty would then be undertaken only if blood pressure remained uncontrollable or if renal function deteriorated.

ACKNOWLEDGEMENTS

We thank Angela McKay for typing the manuscript and Drs J.J. Brown, C.G. Isles and G.W. Herd, MRC Blood Pressure Unit, Western Infirmary, Glasgow, for their help in preparation of this article. We also thank the late Dr T.A.S. Buist and Dr J. Reid, Department of Radiology, Edinburgh Royal Infirmary.

References

1. Genest, J., Cartier, P., Roy, P., Lefebvre, R., Kuchel, O., Cantin, M. and Hammet, P. (1983). Renovascular hypertension. In Genest, J., Kuchel, O., Hammet, P., Cantin, M. (Eds.) *Hypertension*, pp. 1007–1034 (New York: McGraw-Hill)
2. Hodsman, G.P., Brown, J.J., Cumming, A.M.M., Davies, D.L., East, B.W., Lever, A.F., Morton, J.J., Murray, G.D. and Robertson, J.I.S. (1984). Enalapril in treatment of hypertension with renal artery stenosis: changes in blood pressure, renin, angiotensin I and II, renal function and body composition. *Am. J. Med.*, **77** (Suppl. 2A), 52–60
3. Hodsman, G.P. and Robertson, J.I.S. (1983). Captopril: Five years on. *Br. Med. J.*, **287**, 851–2
4. Tillman, D.M., Malatino, L.S., Cumming, A.M.M., Hodsman, G.P., Leckie, B.J., Lever, A.F., Morton, J.J., Webb, D.J. and Robertson, J.I.S. (1984). Enalapril in hypertension with renal artery stenosis: longterm follow-up and effects on renal function. *J. Hypertension*, **2**, (Suppl. 2) 93–100
5. Sos, T.A., Saddekni, S., Pickering, T.G. and Laragh, J.H. (1986). Technical aspects of percutaneous transluminal angioplasty in renovascular disease. *Nephron*, **44** (Suppl. 1), 45–50
6. Hricik, D.E., Browning, P.J., Kopelman, R., Goorno, W.E., Madias, N.E. and

Dzau, V.J. (1983). Captopril-induced functional renal insufficiency in patients with bilateral renal-artery stenoses or renal-artery stenosis in a solitary kidney. *N. Engl. J. Med.*, **308**, 373-6

7. Blythe, W.B. (1983). Captopril and renal autoregulation. *N. Engl. J. Med.*, **308**, 390-1

8. Foster, J.H., Maxwell, M.H., Franklin, S.S., Bleifer, K.H., Trippel, O.H., Julian, O.C., de Camp, P.T. and Varady, P.D. (1975). Renovascular occlusive disease: results of operative treatment. *J. Am. Med. Assoc.*, **231**, 1043-8

9. Franklin, S.S., Young, J.D., Maxwell, M.H., Foster, J.H., Palmer, J.M., Cerny, J. and Varaday, P.D. (1975). Operative morbidity and mortality in renovascular disease. *J. Am. Med. Assoc.*, **231**, 1148-53

10. MacKay A., Boyle, P., Brown, J.J., Cumming, A.M.M., Forrest, H., Graham, A.G., Lever, A.F., Robertson, J.I.S. and Semple, P.F. (1983). The decision on surgery in renal artery stenosis. *Q. J. Med.* **207**, 363-81

11. Sellars, L., Siamopoulos, K., Hacking, P.M., Proud, G., Taylor, R.M.R., Essenhigh, D.M. and Wilkinson, R. (1985). Renovascular hypertension: Ten years' experience in a regional centre. *Q. J. Med.*, **219**, 403-16

12. Sellars, L., Shore, A.C. and Wilkinson, R. (1985). Renal vein renin studies in renovascular hypertension – Do they really help? *J. Hypertension*, **3**, 177-81

13. Gruntzig, A., Kuhlmann, U., Vetter, W., Lutolf, V., Meier, B. and Siegenthaler, W. (1978). Treatment of renovascular hypertension with percutaneous transluminal dilatation of a renal artery stenosis. *Lancet*, **1**, 801-2

14. Geyskes, G.G., Puylaert, C.B.A.J., Oei, H.Y. and Mees, E.J.D. (1983). Follow-up study of 70 patients with renal artery stenosis treated by percutaneous transluminal dilatation. *Br. Med. J.*, **287**, 333-6

15. Colapinto, R.F., Stronell, R.D., Harries-Jones, E.P., Gildiner, M., Hobbs, B.B., Farrow, G.A., Wilson, D.R., Morrow, J.D., Logan, A.G. and Birch, S.J. (1982). Percutaneous transluminal dilatation of the renal artery: follow-up studies on renovascular hypertension. *Am. J. Roentgenol.*, **139**, 727-32

16. Sos, T.A., Pickering, T.G., Sniderman, K., Saddekni, S., Case, D.B., Silane, M.F., Vaughan, E.D. and Laragh, J.H. (1983). Percutaneous transluminal renal angioplasty in renovascular hypertension due to atheroma or fibromuscular dysplasia. *N. Engl. J. Med.*, **309**, 274-9

17. Martin, E.C., Mattern, R.F., Baer, L., Fankuchen, E.I. and Casarella, W.J. (1981). Renal angioplasty for hypertension: predictive factors for longterm success. *Am. J. Roentgenol*, **137**, 921-4

18. Tegtmeyer, C.J., Kofler, T.J. and Ayers, C.A. (1984). Renal angioplasty: current status. *Am. J. Roentgenol.*, **142**, 17-21

19. Atkinson, A.B. and Kellett, R.J. (1974). Value of intravenous urography in investigating hypertension. *J. R. Coll. Physicians. London*, **8** (Suppl. 2), 175-81

20. MacKay, A., Brown, J.J., Lever, A.F., Morton, J.J. and Robertson, J.I.S. (1983). Unilateral renal disease in hypertension. In Robertson J.I.S. (Ed.) *Handbook of Hypertension, Vol. 2, Clinical Aspects of Secondary Hypertension*, pp. 33-97 (Amsterdam: Elsevier)

21. Bookstein, J.J., Abrams, H.L., Buenger, R.E., Lecky, J., Franklin, S.S., Reiss, M.D., Bleifer, K.H., Klatte, E.C., Varaday, P.D. and Maxwell, M.H. (1972). Radiologic aspects of renovascular hypertension. II. The role of urography in unilateral renovascular disease. *J. Am. Med. Assoc.*, **220**, 1225-30

22. Harvey, R.J., Krumlovsky, F., del Greco, F. and Martin H.G. (1985). Is renal

digital subtraction angiography the preferred non invasive test? *J. Am. Med. Assoc.*, **254**, 388–93

23. Maxwell, M.H., Lupu, A.N. and Taplin, G.V. (1968). Radioisotope renogram in renal arterial hypertension. *J. Urol.*, **100**, 376–83

24. MacKay, A., Eadie, A.S., Cumming, A.M.M., Graham, A.G., Adams, F.G. and Horton, P.W. (1981). Assessment of total and divided renal plasma flow by ^{123}I-hippuran renography. *Kidney Int.*, **19**, 49–57

25. Bratt, C.G., Larsson, I. and White, I. (1981). Scintillation camera renography with ^{99M}Tc-DTPA and ^{131}I-hippuran. *Scand. J. Clin. Lab. Invest.*, **41**, 189–97

26. Pors Nielsen, S., Lehd Moller M. and Trap-Jensen, J. (1977). ^{99M}Tc-DTPA scintillation camera renography: a new method for estimation of single kidney function. *J. Nucl. Med.*, **18**, 112–17

27. Wenting, G.J., Tan-Tjiong, H., Derkx, F.H.M., De Bruyn, J.H.B., Man Int Veld, A.J. and Schalekamp, M.A.D.H. (1984). Split renal function after captopril in unilateral renal artery stenosis. *Br. J. Med.*, **288**, 886–90

28. Geyskes, G.G., Oei, H.Y. and Faber, J.A.J. (1986). Renography: prediction of blood pressure after dilatation of renal artery stenosis. *Nephron*, **44** (Suppl. 1), 54–9

29. Sfakianakis, G.N., Bourgoignie, J.J. and Jaffe, D. (1987). The effect of captopril on renography in renovascular hypertension (RVH): a predictor of response to angioplasty (Abstract). *J. Nucl. Med.,* **28** (Suppl.), 613

30. Fommei, E., Ghione, S., Palla, L., Bertelli, P., Marabotti, C. and Palombo, C. (1987). The scintigraphic captopril test in renovascular hypertension (Abstract). *J. Nucl. Med.,* **28** (Suppl.), 613

31. Phillips, D.J., Powers, J.E., Eyers, M.K., Blackshear, W.M., Bodily, K.C., Strandness, D.E. and Baker, D.W. (1980). Detection of peripheral vascular disease using the duplex scanner III. *Ultrasound Med. Biol.*, **6**, 205–18

32. Blackshear, W.M., Phillips, D.J., Chikos, P.M., Hartley, J.D., Thiele, B.L. and Strandness, D.E. (1980). Carotid artery velocity patterns in normal and stenotic vessels. *Stroke*, **11**, 67–71

33. Avasthi, P.S., Voyles, W.F. and Greene, E.R. (1984). Noninvasive diagnosis of renal artery stenosis by echo-Doppler velocimetry. *Kidney Int.*, **25**, 824–9

34. Jenni, R., Vieli, A., Luscher, Th. F., Schneider, E., Vetter, W. and Anliker, M. (1986). Combined two-dimensional ultrasound Doppler technique. New possibilities for the screening of renovascular and parenchymatous hypertension. *Nephron*, **44** (Suppl. 1), 2–4

35. Hillman, B.J., Ovitt, T.W., Nudelman, S., Fisher, H.D., Frost, M.M., Capp, M.P., Roehrig, H. and Seely, G. (1981). Digital video subtraction angiography of renal vascular abnormalities. *Radiology*, **139**, 277–80

36. Osborne, R.W. Jnr., Goldstone, J., Hillman, B.J., Ovitt, T.W., Malone, J.M. and Nudelman, S. (1981). Digital video subtraction angiography: screening technique for renovascular hypertension. *Surgery*, **90**, 932–9

37. Vaughan, E.D. (1985). Renovascular hypertension. Nephrology Forum. *Kidney Int.*, **27**, 811–27

38. Eyler, W.R., Clark, M.D., Garman, J.E., Rian, R.L. and Meininger, D.E. (1962). Angiography of the renal areas including a comparative study of renal arterial stenosis in patients with and without hypertension. *Radiology*, **78**, 879–92

39. Holley, K.E., Hunt, J.C., Brown, A.L., Kincaid, O.W. and Sheps, S.G. (1964).

Renal artery stenosis: a clinical-pathologic study in normotensive patients. *Am. J. Med.*, **37**, 14–22

40. Brown, J.J., Cuesta, V., Davies, D.L., Lever, A.F., Morton, J.J., Padfield, P.L., Robertson, J.I.S., Trust, P., Bianchi, G. and Schalekamp, M.A.D.H. (1976). Mechanisms of renal hypertension. *Lancet*, **1**, 1219–21

41. Luscher, T.F., Greminger, P., Kuhlmann, U., Siegenthaler, W., Largiader, F. and Vetter, W. (1986). Renal venous renin determinations in renovascular hypertension: diagnostic and prognostic value in unilateral renal artery stenosis treated by surgery or percutaneous transluminal angioplasty. *Nephron*, **44** (Suppl. 1), 17–24

42. Maxwell, M.H. (1981). Diagnosis of renovascular hypertension. In Zurukzoglu, W., Pamidimitriou, M., Pyrapasopoulos, Y., Sion, M. and Zamboulins, C. (Eds.) *Proceedings of the 8th International Congress of Nephrology*, pp. 1119–24. Basel: Karger

43. Miller, G.A., Ford, K.K., Braun, S.D., Newman, G.E., Moore, A.V., Jr., Malone, R. and Dunnick, N.R. (1985). Percutaneous transluminal angioplasty *vs* surgery for renovascular hypertension. *Am. J. Roentgenol.*, **144**, 447–50

44. Judson, W.E. and Helmer, O.M. (1965). Diagnostic and prognostic values of renin activity in renal venous plasma in renovascular hypertension. *Hypertension*, **13**, 79–89

45. Brown, J.J., Lever, A.F. and Robertson, J.I.S. (1979). Renal hypertension: aetiology, diagnosis and treatment. In Black Sir D, Jones, N.F. (Eds.) *Renal Disease*, 4th Edn, p. 731, Oxford, Blackwell

46. Michelakis, A.M. and Simmons, J. (1969). Effects of posture on renal vein renin activity in hypertension: its implications in the management of patients with renovascular hypertension. *J. Am. Med. Assoc.*, **208**, 659–62

47. Strong, C.G., Hunt, J.C., Sheps, S.G., Tucker, R.M. and Bernatz, P.E. (1971). Renal venous renin activity: enhancement of sensitivity of lateralisation by sodium depletion. *Am. J. Cardiol.*, **27**, 602–11

48. Mannick, J.A., Huvos, A. and Hollander, W.E. (1969). Post-hydralazine renin release in the diagnosis of renovascular hypertension. *Ann. Surg.*, **170**, 409–15

49. Lyons, D.F., Streck, W.F., Kem, D.C., Brown, R.D., Galloway, D.C., Williams, G.R., Chrysant, S.G., Danisa, K. and Carollo, M. (1983). Captopril stimulation of differential renins in renovascular hypertension. *Hypertension*, **5**, 615–22

50. Marks, L.S. and Maxwell, M.H. (1975). Renal vein renin: value and limitations in the prediction of operative results. *Urol. Clin. N. Am.*, **2**, 311–25

51. Kuhlmann, U., Greminger, P., Gruntzig, A., Schneider, E., Pouliadis, G., Luscher, T., Steurer, J., Siegenthaler, W. and Vetter, W. (1985). Long term experience in percutaneous transluminal dilatation of renal artery stenosis. *Am. J. Med.*, **79**, 692–8

52. Stockigt, J.R., Collins, R.D., Noakes, C.A., Schambelan, M. and Biglieri, E.G. (1972). Renal vein renin in various forms of renal hypertension. *Lancet*, **1**, 1194–8

53. Vaughan, E.D., Buhler, F.R., Laragh, J.H., Sealey, J.E., Baer, L. and Bard, R.H. (1973). Renovascular hypertension: renin measurements to indicate hypersecretion and contralateral suppression, estimate renal plasma flow, and score for surgical curability. *Am. J. Med.*, **55**, 402–14

54. Pickering, T.G., Sos, T.A., Vaughan, E.D., Case, D.B., Sealey, J.E., Harshfield, G.A. and Laragh, J.H. (1984). Predictive value and changes of renin secretion in

hypertensive patients with unilateral renovascular disease undergoing successful renal angioplasty. *Am. J. Med.*, **76**, 398–404

55. Pickering, T.G., Sos, T.A., Vaughan, E.D. and Laragh, J.H. (1986). Differing patterns of renal vein renin secretion in patients with renovascular hypertension, and their role in predicting the response to angioplasty. *Nephron*, **44** (Suppl. 1), 8–11

56. Brunner, H.R., Gavras, H., Laragh, J.H. and Keenan, R. (1973). Angiotensin-II blockade in man by Sar[1]-Ala[8]-angiotensin II for understanding and treatment of high blood pressure. *Lancet*, **2**, 1045–8

57. Streeten, D.H.P., Anderson, G.H., Freiberg, J.M. and Dalakos, T.G. (1975). Use of an angiotensin II antagonist (Saralasin) in the recognition of 'angiotensinogenic' hypertension. *N. Engl. J. Med.*, **292**, 657–62

58. Krakoff, L.R., Ribeiro, A.B., Gorkin, J.U. and Felton, K.R. (1980). Saralasin infusion in screening patients for renovascular hypertension. *Am. J. Cardiol.*, **45**, 609–13

59. Atkinson, A.B., Brown, J.J., Cumming, A.M.M., Fraser, R., Lever, A.F., Leckie, B.J., Morton, J.J. and Robertson, J.I.S. (1982). Captopril in the management of hypertension with renal artery stenosis: its long-term effect as a predictor of surgical outcome. *Am. J. Cardiol.*, **49**, 1460–6

60. Staessen, J., Bulpitt, C., Fagard, R., Lijnen, P. and Amery, A. (1983). Long-term converting-enzyme inhibitor as a guide to surgical curability of hypertension associated with renovascular disease. *Am. J. Cardiol.*, **51**, 1317–22

61. Vaughan, E.D., Case, D.B., Pickering, T.G., Sosa, R.E., Sos, T.A. and Laragh, J.H. (1984). Clinical evaluation of renovascular hypertension and therapeutic decisions. *Urol. Clin. N. Am.*, **11**, 393–407

62. Grim, C.E., Yune, H.Y., Donohue, J.P., Weinberger, M.H., Dilley, R. and Klatte, E.C. (1986). Renal vascular hypertension: surgery *vs.* dilatation. *Nephron*, **44** (Suppl. 1), 96–100

63. Dotter, C.T. and Judkins, M.P. (1964). Transluminal treatment of arteriosclerotic obstruction: description of a new technic and a preliminary report of its application. *Circulation*, **30**, 654–70

64. Gruntzig, A. and Hopff, H. (1974). Perkutane rekanalisation chronischer arterieller Verschlusse mit einem neuen Dilatationskatheter. Modifikation der Dotter-Technik. *Dtsch. Med. Wochenschr.*, **99**, 2502–5

65. Schwarten, D.E. (1980). Transluminal angioplasty of renal artery stenosis: 70 experiences. *Am. J. Roentgenol.*, **135**, 969–74

66. Tegtmeyer, C.J., Ayers, C.A. and Wellons, H.A. (1980). The axillary approach to percutaneous renal artery dilatation. *Radiology*, **135**, 775–6

67. Castaneda-Zuniga, W.R., Formanek, A., Tadavarthy, M., Vlodaver, Z., Edwards, J.E., Zollikofer, C. and Amplatz, K. (1980). The mechanism of balloon angioplasty. *Radiology*, **135**, 565–71

68. Wolf, G.L., Le Veen, R.F. and Ring, E.J. (1984). Potential mechanisms of angioplasty. *Cardiovasc. Intervent. Radiol.*, **7**, 11–17

69. Circuto, K.P., McLean, G.K., Oleaga, J.A., Freiman, D.B., Grossman, R.A. and Ring, E.J. (1981). Renal artery stenosis: anatomic classification for percutaneous angioplasty. *Am. J. Roentgenol.*, **137**, 599–601

70. Flechner, S.M. (1984). Percutaneous transluminal dilatation: a realistic appraisal in patients with stenosing lesions of the renal artery. *Urol. Clin. N. Am.*, **11**, 515–27

71. Sniderman, K.W. and Sos, T.A. (1982). Percutaneous transluminal recanalisation and dilatation of totally occluded renal arteries. *Radiology*, **142**, 607–10

72. Mahler, F., Triller, J., Weidmann, P. and Nachbur, B. (1986). Complications in percutaneous transluminal dilatation of renal arteries. *Nephron*, **44** (Suppl. 1), 60–3

73. Madias, N.E., Ball, J.T. and Millan, V.G. (1981). Percutaneous transluminal renal angioplasty in the treatment of unilateral atherosclerotic renovascular hypertension. *Am. J. Med.*, **70**, 1078–84

74. Millan, V.G., McCauley, J., Kopelman, R.I. and Madias, N.E. (1985). Percutaneous transluminal renal angioplasty in nonatherosclerotic renovascular hypertension: long-term results. *Hypertension*, **7**, 668–74

75. Grim, C.E., Luft, F.C., Yune, H.Y., Klatte, E.C. and Weinberger, M.H. (1981). Percutaneous transluminal dilatation in the treatment of renal vascular hypertension. *Ann. Intern. Med.*, **95**, 439–42

76. Kremer Hovinga, T.K., de Jong, P.E., de Zeeuw, D., Donker, A.J.M., Schuur, K.H. and van der Hem, G.K. (1986). Restenosis prevalence and long-term effects on renal function after percutaneous transluminal renal angioplasty. *Nephron*, **44** (Suppl. 1), 64–7

77. Tegtmeyer, C.J., Kellum, C.D. and Ayers, C. (1984). Percutaneous transluminal angioplasty of the renal artery: results and long-term follow-up. *Radiology*, **153**, 77–84

78. de Jong, P.E., de Zeeuw, D., Smit, A.J., Hoorntjest, S.J., Schuur, K.H., Donker, A.J. and Van der Hem, G.K. (1983). The effect of transluminal dilatation of stenosed renal arteries on kidney function. *Neth. J. Med.*, **26**, 266–70

79. Maxwell, M.H., Bleifer, K.H., Franklin, S.S. and Varaday, P.D. (1972). Cooperative study of renovascular hypertension: demographic analysis of the study. *J. Am. Med. Assoc.*, **220**, 1195–2004

80. Meaney, T.F., Dustan, H.P. and McCormack, L.J. (1968). Natural history of renal arterial disease. *Radiology*, **9**, 877–87

81. Wollenweber, J., Sheps, S.G. and David, D.G. (1968). Clinical course of atherosclerotic renovascular disease. *Am. J. Cardiol.*, **21**, 60–71

82. Schreiber, M.J., Pohl, M.A. and Novick, A.C. (1984). The natural history of atherosclerotic and fibrous renal artery disease. *Urol. Clin. North. Am.*, **11**, 383–92

83. Pickering, T.G., Sos, T.A., Saddekni, S., Rozenblit, G., James, G.D., Orenstein, A., Helseth, G. and Laragh, J.H. (1986). Renal angioplasty in patients with azotaemia and renovascular hypertension. *J. Hypertension*, **4** (Suppl. 6), S667–9

84. Weinberger, M.H., Grim, C.E., Luft, F.C. and Yune, H.Y. (1986). Percutaneous transluminal angioplasty in complicated renal vascular hypertension. *Nephron*, **44** (Suppl. 1), 51–3

85. Lacombe, M. (1975). Arterial stenosis complicating renal allotransplantation in man: a study of thirty-eight cases. *Ann. Surg.*, **181**, 283–8

86. Sagalogsky, A.I. and Peters, P.C. (1984). Renovascular hypertension following renal transplantation. *Urol. Clin. North Am.*, **11**, 491–502

87. Whelton, P.K., Russell, R.P., Harrington, D.P., Williams, G.M. and Walker, W.G. (1979). Hypertension following renal transplantation: causative factors and therapeutic implications. *J. Am. Med. Assoc.*, **241**, 1128–31

88. Flechner, S.M., Sandler, C.M., Childs, T., Ben-Menachem, Y., Van Buren, C., Payne, W. and Kahan, B.D. (1983). Screening for transplant renal artery stenosis in hypertensive recipients using digital subtraction angiography. *J. Urol.*, **130**, 440–4

89. Smith, R.B. and Elrich, R.M. (1976). The surgical complications of renal transplantation. *Urol. Clin. North. Am.*, **3**, 621–46

90. Smith, R.B. Arterial stenosis in renal transplantation. In Kaufmann, J.J. (Ed.) *Current Urologic Therapy*, pp. 151–153. (Philadelphia: W.B. Saunders)

91. Buist, T.A. (1985). Percutaneous renal angioplasty. *J. R. Soc. Med.*, **78**, 353–5

92. Sniderman, K.W., Sos, T.A., Sprayregan, S., Saddekni, S., Cheigh, J.S., Tapia, L., Tellis, V. and Veith, F. (1980). Percutaneous transluminal angioplasty in renal transplant arterial stenosis for relief of hypertension. *Radiology*, **135**, 23–6

93. Mollenkopf, F., Matas, A., Veith, F., Sprayregan, S., Soberman, R. Kuemmel, P., Tellis, V., Sniderman, K.W., Sos, T.A., Cheigh, J.S. and Stubenbord, W. (1983). Percutaneous transluminal angioplasty for transplant renal artery stenosis. *Transplant. Proc.*, **15**, 1089–91

94. Dafoe, D.C., Schoenfeld, R.B. and Grossman, R.A. (1982). Percutaneous transluminal angioplasty treatment of renal allograft artery stenosis. Presented at the *8th Annual Meeting of the American Society of Transplant Surgeons*, Chicago, Illinois, June 3–4

95. Majeski, J.A. and Munda, R. (1981). Hazard of percutaneous transluminal dilatation in renal transplant arterial stenosis. *Arch. Surg.*, **116**, 1225–6

96. Medina, M., Butt, K., Gordon, D.H., Thanawala, S. and Solomon, N. (1981). A complication of percutaneous transluminal angioplasty in the transplanted kidney. *Urol. Radiol.*, **3**, 59

97. Rientgen, D., Van Moore, A., Vernon, W. *et al.* (1983). Percutaneous renal artery angioplasty for transplant renal artery stenosis. *Proc. Am. Soc. Transplant Surg.*, Chicago, Illinois

98. Millar, J.A., Leckie, B.J., Semple, P.F., Morton, J.J., Sonkodi, S. and Robertson, J.I.S. (1978). Active and inactive renin in human plasma: renal arteriovenous differences and relationships with angiotensin and renin substrate. *Circ. Res.*, **43** (Suppl. 1), 120–7

99. Mahler, F., Probst, P., Haertel, M., Weidmann, P. and Krneta, A. (1982). Lasting improvement of renovascular hypertension by transluminal dilatation of atherosclerotic and nonatherosclerotic renal artery stenosis: a follow-up study. *Circulation*, **65**, 611–17

100. Bell, G.M., Reid, J. and Buist, T.A.S. (1987). Percutaneous transluminal angioplasty improves blood pressure and renal function in renovascular hypertension. *Q. J. Med.*, **241**, 393–403

5

HYPERTENSION FOLLOWING RENAL TRANSPLANTATION

R. WILKINSON

DIFFICULTIES IN THE DEFINITION OF HYPERTENSION

Since blood pressure in transplant recipients, as in the general population, is a continuous variable with an approximately Gaussian distribution, any definition of hypertension is, of necessity, arbitrary. In essential hypertension, the problem of definition has been solved by a pragmatic definition: 'The level of blood pressure at which treatment does more good than harm'. This approach is not open to us in the case of the hypertension of patients undergoing treatment for end-stage renal disease, since controlled trials of treatment of hypertension have not been performed, and are never likely to be performed, because of logistical and ethical considerations. Faced with this, nephrologists have not simply adopted the definition derived from trials in essential hypertension for use in renal patients, but rather have tended to be more aggressive in their approach because of the suggestion that careful control of blood pressure may protect against progressive renal damage as well as any effect it may have in reducing vascular disease. Thus, in the majority of studies of transplant recipients, patients have been considered to be hypertensive if the diastolic pressure was 90 mmHg or greater without antihypertensive therapy on three occasions. A more useful approach to defining the extent of the problem, however, is to by-pass the problem of definition on the basis of an arbitrary level and instead describe the distribution of blood pressures observed.

159

PREVALENCE OF HYPERTENSION FOLLOWING TRANSPLANTATION

The reported prevalence varies depending on the definition used, but the distribution of diastolic pressures is generally agreed to be of the following order: 50% less than 90 mmHg, 30% between 90 and 100 mmHg, 17% between 100 and 120 mmHg and 3% greater than 120 mmHg[1,2]. The prevalence of hypertension appears to remain constant on follow-up for as long as 11 years[3]. In children, the prevalence of hypertension appears to be even higher[4], with 86% of recipients hypertensive at one month following transplantation, although this high level may subsequently fall[5] to around 60%.

VASCULAR DISEASE IN TRANSPLANT RECIPIENTS

Despite steady improvement in dialysis and transplantation techniques, the death rate in patients undergoing renal replacement therapy continues to exceed that in the general population[6]. Approximately 40% of deaths in adults below and above the age of 65 years are due to cardiovascular disease[7]. Although it has been argued that much of the vascular damage that subsequently gives rise to myocardial infarction and stroke may develop during the predialysis phase of end-stage renal disease[8], it seems likely from experience in the secondary prevention of myocardial infarction and stroke in non-renal patients that modification of known risk factors for vascular disease in dialysis and transplant patients would be worthwhile. There are, of course, many factors that may be implicated in the accelerated atherosclerosis seen in renal patients. Most of these, including cigarette smoking, which tends to be encouraged by the boredom of dialysis and the unemployment that may go with it, hyperlipidaemia, carbohydrate intolerance, hyperuricaemia, hyperparathyroidism and hyperoxalaemia, which may contribute to vascular calcification, and corticosteroid therapy, are beyond the scope of this chapter, which will concentrate on the role of hypertension in vascular disease.

The role of hypertension in the vascular disease of transplant recipients

There is no dispute over the importance of and need for treatment of severe hypertension in transplant recipients since, especially in children, it may result in hypertensive encephalopathy[4] or heart failure. It is more difficult in the case of mild or moderate hypertension to establish either a causal role in vascular disease or the benefit from treatment. It is unlikely that the longitudinal studies of the natural history of mild hypertension that led to the appreciation of its role in vascular disease in the general population[9] could ever be undertaken in renal disease. Furthermore, a controlled trial of the effectiveness of treatment of mild hypertension in the prevention of vascular disease comparable to the U.K. MRC trial (1985)[10] would not be possible in renal disease, because of the comparatively small number of patients available for inclusion and their variable renal state over the period for which follow-up would be necessary.

In the absence of such direct evidence, it seems reasonable to extrapolate from the data available from the study of essential hypertension in our approach to hypertension in transplant recipients, and to assume that raised blood pressure is a risk factor for vascular disease and that control may improve prognosis.

THE PATHOGENESIS OF RENAL TRANSPLANT HYPERTENSION

Whereas it is unusual to find a surgically correctable cause for hypertension in patients without renal failure, the majority of whom suffer from essential hypertension, the situation might be expected to differ in transplant recipients. Several conditions prevail in these patients (Table 5.1), each of which on its own could cause hypertension; if the factor responsible for the hypertension in a particular individual could be identified then corrective measures might be possible. An understanding of the pathogenesis of hypertension in renal transplant patients is therefore potentially of value in clinical management.

The diversity of the causes of hypertension in transplant recipients makes it unlikely that studies of hormonal and haemodynamic changes will reveal the same pattern in all patients but, taken with the clinical

TABLE 5.1 Factors that may influence blood pressure in renal transplant recipients

Factor	Presumed mechanism
Native kidneys	Renin
Donor kidney	Sodium (?)
Transplant artery stenosis	Renin + sodium
Rejection	Impaired renal function
Acute tubular necrosis	
Dietary sodium	Sodium retention
Corticosteroids	Sodium retention (?)
Cyclosporin	Renal vasoconstriction (?)
Intrarenal arteriovenous fistulae	Renin

features, such studies might be expected to help clarify the mechanism of hypertension in an individual.

The role of elevation of plasma renin in transplant hypertension

In research studies, the measurement of peripheral plasma renin activity has been of value in establishing the role of the native kidneys in transplant hypertension[11,12] and of renin in the hypertension that may accompany acute rejection[13,14]. However, as a practical tool for detecting renin-dependent hypertension, whether due to native kidneys or transplant renal artery stenosis, or as a test for acute rejection, it has been found to be of no value. Plasma renin may be normal in patients with transplant renal artery stenosis[15] and elevated in the absence of stenosis, and it is only inconsistently raised in acute rejection. In practice, therefore, peripheral renin measurements are not employed in the investigation of transplant hypertension.

The role of the host kidneys

There is now good evidence from a number of different approaches that the host kidneys are the major cause of hypertension in a proportion of transplant recipients.

162

Pre-transplant blood pressure and type of renal disease

McHugh *et al.*[12] found a positive correlation between pre- and post-transplant blood pressures in patients not subjected to bilateral nephrectomy, suggesting a role for the host kidneys, although, of course, it could be argued that the hypertension was perpetuated by some non-renal mechanism. In support of the involvement of the native kidneys, however, there are reports that hypertension is more common after transplant in patients whose original disease was glomerulonephritis than in those with structural lesions[4] or interstitial nephritis[16]. It must be added that other groups have not been able to relate post-transplant hypertension to the original renal disease[2,3,17].

Bilateral nephrectomy

Further, more direct support for the importance of the host kidneys comes from the observation that hypertension is much less common in patients who have been subjected to bilateral nephrectomy[3,12,16,18,19] and is frequently improved by bilateral nephrectomy at the time of[20], or after[18,21] transplantation[2].

Plasma renin levels

The presence of the transplanted kidney makes renin measurements difficult to interpret. It seems probable, however, that the host kidneys raise blood pressure through hypersecretion of renin. McHugh *et al.*[12] noted that the plasma renin activity (PRA) was lower in patients who had undergone bilateral nephrectomy and who were usually normotensive, and that blood pressure fell during the infusion of the angiotensin II antagonist saralasin in proportion to the pre-infusion PRA level. This view is not universal, since in some patients hypersecretion of renin by the host kidneys has not been demonstrable (see below) and the presence of a non-renin pressor substance 'nephrotensin' has been suggested as an explanation of the hypertension[22]. The host kidneys are not, of course, the only cause of hypertension in renal transplant recipients, and Wauthier et al.[3] estimate that they are responsible in only about 25% of non-nephrectomized patients.

THE ROLE OF BILATERAL NEPHRECTOMY IN RENAL TRANSPLANTATION

In the past, bilateral nephrectomy was a part of the routine pre-transplant preparation. It became clear, however, that the operation was associated with definite morbidity and even mortality[23], especially in older patients. Yarimizu et al.[24] reported an operative mortality of 11% in patients over the age of 50 years and major morbidity in a further 18%. Pretransplant nephrectomy also led to an exacerbation of anaemia and bone disease that became a major problem for patients who had to wait several years for transplantation. These latter problems may now be partially solved with the availability of 1-α-hydroxy-cholecalciferol, calcitriol, and more recently, erythropoietin[25]. In addition, with better preoperative preparation, surgical risks are certainly less, so that a greater readiness to resort to nephrectomy may develop in the future. One solution to the problems that arose in the anephric patient on dialysis was to undertake nephrectomy at the time of transplantation. Turner et al.[20] reported a mortality of 16% in 38 patients subjected to this procedure, but 5 of the 6 deaths were from sepsis and some of the patients had also been subjected to splenectomy, which Rai et al.[26] have previously shown to be associated with increased mortality.

Prediction of response to bilateral nephrectomy

In view of the problems associated with bilateral nephrectomy and with the availability of better drug therapy, the operation is now rarely undertaken for hypertension. There remain a few patients, however, in whom hypertension cannot be controlled with drugs and for whom bilateral nephrectomy is considered. Since nephrectomy is not always effective in lowering blood pressure, means of predicting the likely response to surgery have been sought. McHugh et al.[12] have found a trend towards increased peripheral vein plasma renin activity in hypertensive transplant recipients, but this did not reach statistical significance and as there was a considerable overlap between normotensive and hypertensive patients, it was not considered to be of value in selecting patients for nephrectomy. Coles *et al.*[21] also found that response to nephrectomy bore no relationship to plasma renin concentration. It has been suggested that the response to captopril may be useful in selecting patients for nephrectomy[27]; this, however, remains to be proved and it seems unlikely that it will be any more specific than the level of PRA, which it tends to mirror.

Measurement of renal vein renin from the native and transplanted kidneys would seem to be the most direct approach to detecting and localizing any hypersecretion of renin. Early experience suggested that this approach might be useful when the response to nephrectomy was predicted correctly in 3 out of the 4 patients studied[28], and in 3 of 3 subjected to nephrectomy[29]. Khoury *et al.*[30] localized hypersecretion of renin to the native kidneys in 10 of 44 patients studied, but did not proceed to nephrectomy, so that the relevance of the finding is not clear. Most groups have, however, found renal vein renin studies unhelpful because bilateral nephrectomy was sometimes curative even when renin hypersecretion was localized to the graft[2,31,32]. Renal vein renin samples were collected simultaneously from host and graft kidneys by van Ypersele de Strihou *et al.*[31] and renin secretion was stimulated with frusemide by Rao *et al.*[2]. However, no group has combined simultaneous collection of renal vein renin samples from host and graft kidneys with acute renin stimulation by a vasodilator or diuretic to overcome the problem of recirculation of renin (which has a half-life in plasma of approximately 30–45 minutes). It may be, therefore, that with these additional refinements, renal vein sampling might prove to be of value. Nevertheless, these additional techniques are not used in clinical decision-making at present.

Indications for bilateral nephrectomy

Bilateral nephrectomy is undertaken in the rare situations in which blood pressure cannot be controlled by medical treatment, provided that graft function is stable, plasma creatinine is less than 200 μmol/l, and renal angiography has excluded transplant renal artery stenosis.

There are no tests that can reliably predict response to nephrectomy. As the procedure is still accompanied by significant morbidity and occasional mortality, the effectiveness of percutaneous renal embolization in producing infarction has been explored as an alternative.

THERAPEUTIC PERCUTANEOUS RENAL ABLATION

The technique of percutaneous transcatheter embolization has become quite widely used for such purposes as arresting gastrointestinal haemorrhage and bleeding following renal biopsy, infarcting tumours, and thrombosing arteriovenous fistulae. In 1984, the Oxford group[33] reported the results of embolization of the host kidneys in 13 patients with hypertension following renal transplantation. Blood-pressure control was markedly improved in 9 and morbidity was limited to nausea, vomiting and loin pain that lasted for 24–36 hours. Blood pressure was, however, only mildly elevated on medical therapy in the majority of their patients and it has been pointed out that the study included no controls and that blood pressure may fall spontaneously in such subjects[34]. There has been one further report of renal embolization for hypertension in transplant recipients[35]. The kidneys were successfully infarcted, but hypertension recurred in one of the patients following an episode of rejection and one patient suffered a femoral artery occlusion requiring surgical intervention. Both groups demonstrated that complete infarction of the kidneys could be achieved but venous renin activity was reduced in only 4 of the 13 Oxford patients.

The present status of therapeutic embolization is therefore uncertain. It is not without morbidity but does appear safer than nephrectomy. Its efficacy, however, is not yet proven and it should be employed with the same conservative approach as bilateral nephrectomy, being reserved for the patient with severe resistant hypertension. If its use is to be extended to milder hypertensives, who constituted the majority of the Oxford group, then this should be in the context of a clinical trial comparing embolization with continuing medical treatment.

HYPERTENSION CAUSED BY THE DONOR KIDNEY

It has been accepted for some time that hypertension can be induced in normotensive rats by the transplantation of a kidney from a hypertensive strain[36]. In man, the importance of the kidney in determining blood pressure was first demonstrated by Curtis *et al.*[37] who showed that transplantation of kidneys from normotensive donors into recipients with renal failure due to nephrosclerosis caused by essential hypertension resulted in prolonged normotension. These observations, though interesting, fall short of establishing a central role for the transplanted kidney in blood pressure control, since mean follow-up was only 4–5 years and no control group given kidneys from donors known to be hypertensive or from a hypertensive family was studied. Guidi *et al.*[38,39] have, however, reported that transplant recipients from normotensive families were more likely to become hypertensive when receiving kidneys from donors with a family history of hypertension than when the donor came from a normotensive family.

Further support for this concept comes from the observation of Strandgaard and Hansen[40] that recipients of kidneys from donors who died of subarachnoid haemorrhage, and had evidence of hypertension, were more hypertensive than those receiving kidneys from donors dying of head injury or cerebral tumour.

These observations are of great interest and practical relevance. They emphasize the need to continue the practice of avoiding hypertensive donors, whether living related or cadaver. Furthermore, they indicate that it would be best to avoid donors with a family history of hypertension and cadaver donors dying from subarachnoid haemorrhage in case they might be hypertensive. This is, however, a counsel of perfection, since there is a continuing shortage of donors, and patients dying from subarachnoid haemorrhage constitute a major source of organs. A renal transplant with hypertension is probably a better prospect for most dialysis patients than no transplant at all.

TRANSPLANT RENAL ARTERY STENOSIS

Prevalence

The frequency with which transplant artery stenosis is reported depends to a large extent on the vigour with which it is sought. The prevalence reported has varied from 1.5% to 16%[41] when arteriography was performed in patients selected for investigation on clinical grounds, usually because of severe resistant hypertension. The prevalence is, of course, also influenced by surgical technique and might be expected to be lower in large centres where surgeons have greater experience. Perhaps the best estimate of prevalence comes from Nilson, et al.[42] who subjected patients to routine angiography and studied 367 of 419 consecutive grafts (88%) and detected stenosis in 22 (6%). In only 13 of these was the stenosis associated with hypertension, so that the prevalence of significant renal artery stenosis was around 3.5%. This figure is in agreement with that observed in other large series, 5.0% of 239 patients[43], 4.4% of 319 patients[44], 2.7% of 914 transplants[45], 4.9% of 405 grafts[31], and 6.1% of 440 patients[16].

The types and causes of renal artery stenosis

Faenze et al.[41] have classified transplant renal artery stenosis (TRAS) into four types. The stenosis may rarely be in the host's internal iliac artery, when it is probably due to progression of atherosclerosis. Stenosis may occur at the suture line, when it is usually attributed to faulty surgical technique although this is by no means certain. If the internal iliac or donor artery is very long, kinking may occur with angulation stenosis. The most common type of stenosis is characterized by a segmental stenosis usually just distal to the anastomosis and thought to be due to trauma of the donor vessel during cannulation for perfusion or from clamping the renal artery. It has, however, been suggested that this type of stenosis might be a manifestation of rejection, since complement can be demonstrated in the vessel wall[46]. There has been one case report of fibromuscular dysplasia affecting the transplant artery when the donor had an aneurysm affecting the contralateral renal artery and probably had pre-existing fibromuscular dysplasia[47].

Faenza et al.[41] have outlined measures designed to prevent renal artery stenosis. These include avoiding pump preservation and the use of vascular clamps on the renal artery, both of which increase the risk of damage to the graft artery. They also recommend that an end-to-side short arterial anastomosis should be used to avoid kinking and the often-diseased internal iliac artery.

Clinical features of renal artery stenosis after transplantation

Hypertension due to renal artery stenosis usually develops in the first 3–6 months following transplantation[41] but may present much later than this. Tilney et al.[45] found the mean time to onset was 21 months. The hypertension tends to be severe[48] but this might simply reflect the greater tendency to subject patients with severe hypertension to angiography. Renal function may be slightly impaired and it is important to exclude rejection before subjecting patients to procedures to correct a possibly significant renal artery stenosis. The value of the presence of a renal artery bruit in the diagnosis of TRAS is uncertain. Jachuck and Wilkinson[49] found that bruits detected within the first two months following transplantation often disappeared spontaneously, but bruits persisting beyond this time were usually associated with hypertension and renal artery stenosis. However, others have regarded the presence of a vascular bruit simply as a sign of good renal perfusion[50]. There is no doubt that a bruit may be audible in the absence of TRAS; indeed, in one study[44], 25% of patients without stenosis had a bruit. It is also clear from the same study that significant TRAS may exist in the absence of a bruit. Thus the detection of a bruit raises the index of suspicion but is by no means diagnostic of renal artery stenosis.

Anatomical diagnosis of TRAS

This can only be made with confidence by renal arteriography, which has all the risks associated with arterial puncture. Khoury et al.[30] suggested that digital subtraction angiography (DSA), in which the contrast medium is given as an intravenous bolus, might be a useful

169

and safer substitute for direct arteriography and detected 7 stenoses in 65 patients studied. However, as they did not seek to confirm their findings by direct arteriography, the reliability of the technique is uncertain. Flechner *et al.*[51], describing two cases of stenosis detected by DSA and confirmed by catheter angiography, recommended intravenous DSA as a useful screening procedure. This view was supported by Clark and Alexander[52] in a larger study of non-transplant patients in which DSA identified 33 of 37 stenoses detected by conventional angiography but gave less clear images with poor demonstration of secondary and intrarenal arteries. Standard angiography is still necessary before surgical repair, but, of course, intravenous DSA provides a particularly useful method of screening for patients who may be suitable for percutaneous translaminal angioplasty (PTA) which will, in any case, be immediately preceded by standard angiography.

A new approach to the diagnosis of transplant artery stenosis – echo-Doppler velocimetry – has recently been described[53]; it appears to correlate with DSA but requires further evaluation.

Unfortunately, the DTPA renal scan which is useful in the diagnosis of unilateral renal artery stenosis in non-transplant patients is not of value in the diagnosis of TRAS[4] because of the absence of a normal contralateral kidney for comparison. The scan may prove of more value if performed with and without converting enzyme blockade, which reduces glomerular filtration rate in kidneys with stenosis of the renal artery. This is, however, unlikely in the transplant patient, since changes in plasma creatinine concentrations are likely to be just as sensitive, much safer and cheaper.

Functional diagnosis

As for non-transplant patients with renal artery stenosis, the conclusion that the stenosis is functionally significant can only be reached after correction of the stenosis has resulted in cure of the hypertension. Unfortunately, again as in the case of the non-transplant patient, no test exists that reliably predicts response to correction of the stenosis.

Renal vein renin

Renal vein renin studies have appeared promising in some limited studies[32,29], but most groups have found the results unhelpful[31,2]; the situation is similar to that observed in non-transplant renal artery stenosis[54].

Peripheral plasma renin

As has already been discussed in relation to the role of the host kidneys, peripheral plasma renin levels are not of value in the diagnosis of renal artery stenosis in transplant recipients. Kornerup and Pedersen[15] found an increase in mean plasma renin concentration in patients with TRAS, but there was considerably overlap with values found in normotensive and otner hypertensive patients.

Response to converting enzyme blockade

Although it seems unlikely that the hypotensive response to converting enzyme blockade will provide a specific test for renin-dependent hypertension[55], there is some evidence to suggest that its effect on renal function will be of value. Farrow and Wilkinson[56] first described the development of reversible renal failure with captopril in a patient with transplant renal artery stenosis, and it was subsequently suggested that this might arise as a consequence of efferent arteriolar vasodilation as the result of blockade of angiotensin II production[57]. Curtis et al.[55] found that serum creatinine increased following captopril only in patients with TRAS, and van der Woude et al.[58] reported a reduction in glomerular filtration rate (GFR) in all 9 patients with TRAS given the drug. Deterioration in renal function following blockade of angiotensin converting enzyme is therefore strongly suggestive of the presence of significant TRAS. What is less certain, however, is whether the absence of such a deterioration in function can be taken to exclude stenosis. There have been reports of the successful treatment of hypertension associated with TRAS with converting enzyme inhibitors. Trachtman et al.[59], Venkatachalam and Kosanovich[60], and Luke

171

et al.[61] point out that it has not yet been established that maintenance of renal function during converting enzyme blockade excludes functionally significant TRAS. They do, however, describe two patients with stenosis who maintained their GFR when given captopril and did not respond to technically successful angioplasty.

In summary, therefore, deterioration of renal function following converting enzyme blockade suggests the presence of TRAS which is functionally significant, but correction of a stenosis may still be worthwhile even when GFR is maintained during blockade. Renin studies are not of proven value and should be undertaken only as part of a research study. The indications for intervention to correct TRAS are, therefore, hypertension that cannot be controlled satisfactorily, or deteriorating renal function that is not due to rejection. The response to correction cannot be reliably predicted.

The treatment of transplant renal artery stenosis

Before the introduction of percutaneous transluminal angioplasty for renal artery stenosis in 1978, correction of transplant artery stenosis involved major surgery with a considerable risk of graft loss. A conservative approach was therefore adopted in most transplant centres, except for the most resistant hypertensives or cases when graft function was declining. Jachuck *et al.*[43] found that in eight patients with TRAS and severe hypertension, control of blood pressure with drugs was satisfactory and renal function did not deteriorate over more than one year of follow up. Furthermore, there have been reports of spontaneous regression of TRAS in five cases[62-64], lending some support to the case for a conservative approach. The kidney, however, may suffer permanent damage from prolonged ischaemia and there is, therefore, a continuing need to correct stenosis in selected patients. The results of surgical intervention from some centres have been excellent and there are now many reports of successful PTA.

Surgical correction of TRAS

The surgical correction of TRAS is difficult because of dense scar tissue around the transplanted kidney. The discussion of surgical technique is beyond the scope of this chapter, but patch angioplasty with saphenous vein, by-pass grafting with saphenous vein, autogenous artery, or, less commonly, synthetic material, or resection and direct re-anastomosis may be employed[65]. The published results of surgical correction of TRAS have been reviewed by Lohr et al.[66]. Of 180 procedures, 130 (72%) were technically successful, 20 kidneys (11%) were lost and 5 patients (2.8%) died. In seven other reports not included by Lohr, the conclusions have been similar. Of 62 patients in all, 54 operations (87%) were technically successful, only 2 kidneys (3.2%) were lost, mortality was 1.6% and hypertension was cured in 61% and improved in 23%[2,31,41,65,67–69]. It is likely, of course, that published results are better than those generally achieved, since there is a natural tendency to report successful experience. However, it does seem that surgery will be technically successful in about 75% of cases and that hypertension will be cured or improved in about two-thirds of patients. Unfortunately, there is a real risk or graft loss (10%) and mortality (2.5%). This has led to a move towards percutaneous angioplasty as primary treatment.

Percutaneous transluminal angioplasty

Percutaneous transluminal angioplasty (PTA) is now the first approach in non-transplant renal artery stenosis and, since its first use in transplants in 1979[70], it has been gaining a similar place in the management of TRAS. Lohr et al.[66] have reviewed the published reports of the results of PTA. Of 90 procedures reported, 76 (84%) were technically successful and only one graft was lost. In three other reports not included by Lohr[68,67,71], there were 11 patients in all with technical success in 7 (64%) and cure of hypertension in 4 (36%). There were no grafts lost and no deaths. Chandrasoma[67] noted very poor results with angioplasty in four patients with stenosis at the anastomotic site. All had fibrosis and calcification at the site of stenosis and did well with surgical resection. Angioplasty can be successfully repeated when stenosis recurs[72], but repeated attempts after initial failure of the technique are probably not worthwhile[73]. We have come across patients in our own practice in whom dilatation is not possible despite correct positioning of the balloon. This is presumably due to dense fibrosis. There has been one report of renal artery perforation associated with balloon rupture[74], and arterial dissection is also a possibility during the procedure. It is essential, therefore, to have surgical back-up facilities when undertaking angioplasty.

The relative roles of surgery and angioplasty

Angioplasty is safer than surgery and when intervention for renal artery stenosis is indicated (i.e. when blood pressure cannot be controlled by drugs or when renal function is deteriorating) it should be attempted first. It will be unsuccessful in a proportion of patients and surgery will be indicated for some of these. However, as surgery carries the risk of graft loss, and even mortality, the threshold for intervention by angioplasty is lower than for surgery. Early surgical intervention will not be indicated in all cases of failed angioplasty, and a further trial of medical treatment might be worthwhile.

Medical treatment of hypertension due to TRAS

One should initially use standard antihypertensive drugs. The precise drugs to be used are a matter of individual experience and preference, but a common treatment would be β-adreno-receptor antagonist, initially with the subsequent addition of diuretic, calcium antagonist and α-adreno-receptor blocker in sequence. In resistant cases, methyldopa still has a place. In men whose hypertension is resistant to these drugs in various combinations, the potent vasodilator minoxidil usually controls pressure. Large doses of a loop diuretic are usually necessary to counteract the fluid retention that is commonly associated with powerful vasodilators. The use of minoxidil in women is limited by its propensity to cause hirsutism. If renal artery stenosis is known to exist, the converting enzyme inhibitors are usually avoided because of the risk of renal failure. If, however, other drugs are not effective or are unacceptable to the patient, captopril or enalapril may be tried with careful monitoring of renal function.

If blood pressure is easily controlled with drugs and renal function is stable, it is reasonable to continue with medical treatment, since the hazards of intervention are probably greater than the risk of ischaemic fibrosis in the kidney. Poor medical control or deterioration of renal function are clear indications for intervention.

GRAFT FUNCTION AND HYPERTENSION

Renal function tends to be poorer in transplant recipients with hypertension persisting more than 6 months after transplant than in normotensive patients [1-3,16,75]. Hypertensive diabetic transplant recipients appear to fare particularly badly[76]. It is not clear whether the renal failure is the cause or the effect of the hypertension. The observation of Wauthier et al.[3] that at 3 months post-transplant renal function is the same in normotensive and hypertensive patients and that the difference reaches significance only after 7 years, suggests that the renal failure may be secondary to prolonged hypertension. This is perhaps surprising, since deteriorating renal function is rarely seen in non-malignant essential hypertension. Hypertension, however, does seem to accelerate the rate of renal impairment in patients with intrinsic renal disease[77] and this may also be true in patients with a single kidney. On the other hand, the observation that hypertensive patients had suffered more episodes of rejection than the normotensives[16,31] suggests that immunologically-mediated renal damage might be the primary event.

The mechanism by which a mild impairment of renal function might cause hypertension is not clear but will be discussed below.

STEROID DOSE AND HYPERTENSION

It has been generally accepted that high levels of glucocorticoids, whether endogenous as in Cushing's syndrome, or exogenous, are associated with the development of hypertension, although doubt has been cast on whether or not glucocorticoids themselves raise blood pressure[78]. If they do cause hypertension, the mechanism is not clear. It has been suggested that their mild mineralocorticoid activity causing sodium retention might be responsible. Indeed, we have reported a significant increase in total body exchangeable sodium in hypertensive transplant recipients. Their prednisone dosage was also higher than that of the normotensive patients, but the difference did not reach statistical significance[12]. Glucocorticoids increase hepatic synthesis of angiotensinogen and might therefore raise blood pressure by raising plasma renin activity[79].

The relationship of prednisone dose to blood pressure in renal transplant recipients is, however, not clear. Early reports suggested that blood pressure was related to steroid dosage in the first few months after transplantation[13,75]. In addition, Luke et al.[61] reported that higher doses of maintenance steroids were associated with higher systolic and diastolic pressures. The importance of steroids appeared to be supported by the observation that the change from daily to alternate-day prednisone therapy resulted in a reduction in blood pressure[61,79-81]. However, there have now been several reports of a lack of association between steroid dose and hypertension[2,18,21] in patients followed for several years after transplantation.

This, of course, must cast doubt on the importance of prednisone dosage in the range used for long-term immunosuppression in the aetiology of hypertension. Nevertheless, it is possible to reconcile the conflicting observations. The situation is analogous to the role of salt intake in essential hypertension, where dietary sodium does not differ between hypertensive and normotensive patients and yet a reduction in dietary sodium does lower blood pressure. Prednisone may contribute to hypertension only in susceptible individuals and a reduction in dosage or change to alternate-day therapy in these people may result in a fall in blood pressure. Other patients may be able to tolerate large doses of steroid without developing hypertension. Further carefully controlled trials of the value of a change to alternate-day prednisone therapy would be worthwhile.

BODY WEIGHT AND HYPERTENSION

In patients with essential hypertension, weight reduction is accompanied by a reduction in blood pressure[82]. In transplant recipients, body weight increases during the first year. Although the increase occurs in both normotensive and hypertensive patients, it is greater in hypertensives[19] and this difference persists for up to 7 years[31].

It is not known whether the obesity contributes to hypertension in transplant recipients and, if so, by what mechanism. A prospective trial of the effect of weight reduction without any change in other dietary constituents such as alcohol, sodium and calcium will be necessary to determine the exact role of obesity. Until such information becomes available, it seems reasonable to advise calorie restriction in all obese patients but particularly in those who are hypertensive.

SALT INTAKE

There is still considerable debate on the role of sodium intake in the pathogenesis of essential hypertension. The data relating mean sodium intake of a *nation* to the prevalence of hypertension in that country are suspect in it has not so far been possible to relate blood pressures of individuals to their sodium intake within national populations[83]. However, there is indirect support for the role of salt in essential hypertension in that restriction of dietary sodium has been shown to result in some reduction in blood pressure[84].

It has been suggested that in renal transplant recipients increased dietary sodium does not contribute to hypertension. Kalbfleisch *et al.*[85] found a strikingly increased dietary sodium intake in transplant recipients (43% higher than controls), but hypertension was present in less than half, tended to be mild, and was not related to sodium intake. However, many of his patients were taking diuretic drugs that might account for the high sodium intake. Curtis *et al.*[86] showed that, unlike patients with essential hypertension, hypertensive transplant recipients did not vary their blood pressure in response to sodium loading or depletion; this again suggests that sodium intake was not an important determinant of blood pressure. However, the periods on each sodium intake were only 3 or 4 days and it remains possible that the response might be different under more normal circumstances of prolonged dietary exposure to a change in sodium intake. McHugh et al.[12] studied 94 renal transplant recipients in whom all antihypertensive drugs and diuretics had been withdrawn for 2 weeks. Urinary sodium was slightly higher in the hypertensive patients but the difference did not reach statistical significance. In view of differences in individual susceptibility to salt-induced hypertension, it is not surprising that a relationship between sodium intake and hypertension has not been seen in the relatively small numbers of patients included in the studies reported to date. It seems likely that very large numbers of patients will be required to establish or refute such a relationship.

In the absence of firm evidence incriminating dietary sodium, it would seem wise not to recommend severe dietary sodium restriction in hypertensive transplant recipients but, at the same time, reasonable to extrapolate from evidence in essential hypertension and advise against very high sodium intake.

CYCLOSPORIN AND HYPERTENSION

Cyclosporin (CsA) now has an established place in the treatment of patients receiving renal transplants[87,88] Most groups have reported an increased incidence of hypertension in patients treated with CsA[5,87,89,90], although Henny et al.[88], perhaps because they studied smaller numbers, found that the difference in incidence did not reach statistical significance. Chapman and Morris[91], however, found that blood pressure was not higher in CsA-treated than in azathioprine-treated patients at 90 days and actually fell to less than that of the azathioprine group when CsA was withdrawn at 90 days.

In the early stages of treatment, the elevation of blood pressure and reduction in renal function may result from an increase in renal allograft vascular resistance[92], which may be due to an increase in the thromboxane A_2 prostaglandin I_2 ratio[93]. At this stage, the impairment of renal function is completely reversible[88] and blood pressure falls over a period of 1 week following withdrawal of CsA[91].

There is less certainty regarding the consequences of long-term CsA treatment. Irreversible renal damage with renal failure has been reported in heart transplant recipients treated with CsA[94]. The Canadian study[87] identified a subgroup of 29 patients (of 496 studied) who developed renal impairment that required a change from CsA treatment. These patients tended to have longer cold ischaemia and surgical anastomosis times and higher CsA levels in the early post-transplant period. The authors suggested that patients with these adverse features should be given alternative maintenance immuno-suppressive therapy. In the remainder of the patients in the Canadian study, mean serum creatinine concentrations were not strikingly different at 2 years between the CsA group ($202\,\mu$mol/l) and the patients receiving standard therapy ($176\,\mu$mol/l). Henny et al.[88] found that at 1 year renal function was actually better in the CsA-treated than the azathioprine-treated patients. Thus, chronic renal damage resulting from prolonged CsA therapy is a real possibility but is not inevitable if low doses are used and high-risk patients are converted to alternative therapy. Unfortunately, renal histology does not give a clear answer to whether chronic renal damage due to CsA has occurred. Diffuse interstitial fibrosis and cellular infiltration may be seen in patients who have been treated with CsA, but similar changes occur in transplant recipients not given CsA[91]. If renal damage can be avoided, hypertension should not be a problem with long-term CsA therapy and this has been borne out so far by the results of both the Canadian[87] and the Leiden[88] studies.

INTRARENAL ARTERIOVENOUS FISTULAE

Most renal transplant recipients undergo at least one transplant biopsy and intrarenal arteriovenous fistulae are a rare complication of this procedure. In an experience of almost 1000 renal transplants in New-castle, the authors have detected only two patients with this compli-cation. Zinman and Libertino[98] have reviewed the subject thoroughly, outlined the major clinical features, and suggested management. The majority of patients who develop this complication have pre-existing hypertension. Presentation is usually with both haematuria and hyper-tension and many patients have a continuous bruit over the transplant. Diagnosis in transplant patients is usually made at arteriography, although compression and distortion of the collecting system may be seen on intravenous urography. Hypertension, which occurs in about half of the patients, is thought to arise because of renal ischaemia beyond the fistula, due to shunting, with a resultant increase in renin release. It has, however, not been possible to demonstrate an increase in renal vein renin.

The majority of fistulae that complicate renal biopsy close spontaneously and are best treated conservatively. The indications for intervention are continuing heavy haematuria or hypertension that is resistant to medical treatment. We have controlled hypertension successfully with a converting enzyme inhibitor when it had been difficult to control with other drugs. If intervention is required, percutaneous intravascular embolization is the treatment of choice, and when it is carried out by experienced hands the volume of kidney infarcted beyond the fistula may be small. However, this infarct may itself later contribute to hypertension. Similarly, infarction of renal tissue by ligation of a feeding artery or scarring following partial nephrectomy for a polar fistula may perpetuate hypertension if the fistula is treated surgically.

PATHOPHYSIOLOGY OF 'IDIOPATHIC' HYPERTENSION AFTER TRANSPLANTATION

Haemodynamic and hormonal studies have been undertaken predominantly in transplant recipients who were hypertensive but who had no evidence of renal artery stenosis, renal failure, rejection or excessive steroid therapy. Such patients had, in general, stable renal function with plasma creatinine concentrations less than $200 \mu mol/l$, were more than 1 year post-transplant, were on maintenance doses of prednisolone, had no episodes of acute rejection in the previous 3 months, and had no clinical signs to suggest renal artery stenosis.

Cardiac output and peripheral resistance

Cardiac index was similar in hypertensive and normotensive transplant recipients[96,97], so that the difference in blood pressure was due to an increase in peripheral resistance. The mechanism of this increase in resistance is still disputed.

Plasma noradrenaline

Plasma noradrenaline levels have been found to be elevated in renal transplant recipients[96] but the levels are similar in hypertensive and normotensive patients[93,96]. However, Smith et al.[96] noted an increased sensitivity to infused noradrenaline that correlated closely with the blood pressure and which, together with an expansion of body sodium, appeared to account for most of the elevation in blood pressure in their patients.

Plasma renin

Most studies of plasma renin activity or concentration have shown increased levels in renal transplant recipients without evidence of complications[86,96] and studies in which a significant increase has not been demonstrated have usually included only small numbers of patients[98]. There is controversy over whether renin levels are higher in hypertensive than in normotensive patients. Smith and his colleagues[96] found that they were not, and concluded that renin was not responsible for the observed increase in peripheral resistance and could not explain the increased exchangeable sodium in hypertensives. Several other groups, all studying rather small numbers of patients, have also been unable to demonstrate increased renin levels in hypertensives[11,97,99]. However, in a large study, McHugh et al.[12] found a trend towards an increase in PRA in hypertensives and, although this did not reach statistical significance, did observe a reduction in blood pressure in proportion to the level of PRA in response to the infusion of the angiotensin II antagonist saralasin, suggesting an important role for renin in the pathogenesis of the hypertension.

The source of the increased levels of renin is probably the native kidneys, since McHugh et al. and others have found that hypertension is less common in patients who have undergone bilateral nephrectomy. Smith et al.[96], Linas et al.[100], and McHugh et al. have shown that PRA was significantly lower in nephrectomized transplant recipients.

The way in which increased levels of renin might cause hypertension is again uncertain. Whether plasma aldosterone levels are increased in hypertensive patients is disputed and the role of renin in the increased peripheral resistance remains unclear.

Aldosterone

A significant difference in plasma aldosterone concentration between hypertensive and normotensive patients has not been demonstrated; this led Smith et al.[96] to conclude that aldosterone could not be responsible for the increase in exchangeable sodium that they observed. However, urinary aldosterone excretion probably gives a better measure of the physiological activity of aldosterone than can be provided by a single plasma level, and McHugh et al.[12] have found this to be significantly increased in hypertensive patients and to correlate with both blood pressure and PRA.

Exchangeable sodium and blood volume

Kornerup and Pedersen[15] described an increase in total exchangeable sodium (Na_E) in hypertensive transplant recipients who did not have renal artery stenosis. This has been confirmed by McHugh et al.[12] and by Smith et al.[96], who also reported that blood volume was not increased in the hypertensives. Horvath et al.[11] had been unable to demonstrate any difference in extracellular fluid volume (ECFV), plasma volume or blood volume between hypertensive and normotensive patients, but changes in ECFV caused by varying salt intake correlated with changes in blood pressure. Thus, volume changes do seem to be important in determining blood pressure. Smith left the mechanism of the increase in Na_E an open issue because plasma aldosterone levels were normal. McHugh et al.[12] consider that it is likely to be due to the increase in aldosterone secretion, which is in turn due to increased levels of renin, since they found an increase in urinary aldosterone in hypertensive patients and a significant positive correlation between urinary aldosterone and PRA. It remains possible, of course, that aldosterone is not the only reason for the sodium retention that occurs in the hypertensive patients; changes in renal vascular resistance provide an alternative explanation.

Renal vascular resistance

Bennett et al.[101] described a reduction in renal blood flow in hypertensive transplant recipients, but this was largely explained by structural damage to the intrarenal vessels. More recently, Curtis et al.[102] found a striking increase in renal vascular resistance and reduction in renal plasma flow with a less marked reduction in GFR – so that filtration fraction was increased – in hypertensive graft recipients who also had increased PRA. Renal plasma flow was greater in patients who had undergone bilateral nephrectomy[61]; its reduction in patients retaining their original kidneys was shown to be reversible by demonstrating an increase in renal plasma flow with a decrease in PRA following bilateral nephrectomy[102]. It seems likely, therefore, that renin secreted by the host kidneys causes vasoconstriction in the allograft, and this may contribute to the sodium retention that has been observed in hypertensive recipients. The increased filtration fraction suggests that constriction affects predominantly the efferent arteriole, so that proximal tubular reabsorption of sodium will be increased due to a combination of reduced hydrostatic pressure and increased oncotic pressure in the peritubular capillaries.

Summary of proposed pathogenesis of 'idiopathic' post-transplant hypertension

An outline of one possible sequence, including the factors that have been discussed above, is shown in Figure 5.1. The increase in cardiac output arising from the sodium retention is transitory and is followed by an increase in peripheral resistance with return of cardiac output to normal. Two explanations for the transition from high cardiac output to high peripheral resistance have been put forward. The first[103] was that it might be due to all of the vascular beds in the body autoregulating their own blood flow, so that total peripheral resistance increased in response to an increase in cardiac output. The other[104] was that a natriuretic hormone, as yet not isolated, might be released in response to volume expansion and might result in an increase in intracellular sodium and calcium leading to increased vascular tone.

183

PROPOSED PATHOGENESIS OF HYPERTENSION FOLLOWING TRANSPLANT

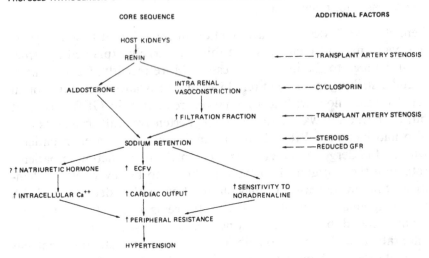

FIGURE 5.1 In patients with an uncomplicated course following transplantation, the host kidneys are probably of central importance in the pathogenesis of hypertension. This hypertension may be exacerbated by the factors on the right of the figure.

PATHOPHYSIOLOGY OF HYPERTENSION IN TRAS

Transplant renal artery stenosis appears to provide the human equivalent of the Goldblatt single-kidney model in which, in the established hypertension phase, PRA is not raised[105], because of suppression by sodium retention[106]. There are certainly many reports of normal or suppressed renin production from the renal allograft in patients with TRAS. There have, however, been reports of increased plasma renin concentration in patients with this condition[15], so that the human situation might not be exactly analogous to the animal model, and renin, possibly derived from the host kidneys, might make an important contribution to hypertension in TRAS.

Measurements of total body exchangeable sodium (Na_E) are difficult to interpret. Correction of TRAS was, however, followed by a fall in Na_E[15], or in body weight[2], suggesting that sodium overload had been present before intervention.

It therefore seems reasonable to conclude that TRAS raises blood pressure through a combination of hypersecretion of renin and sodium overload. These effects will, of course, interact with other factors influencing blood pressure, as shown in the Figure 5.1.

PATHOPHYSIOLOGY OF HYPERTENSION IN PATIENTS WITH MILD IMPAIRMENT OF RENAL FUNCTION

Brod et al.[107,108] found that the first change in patients who had only minimal impairment of renal function but who subsequently developed hypertension, was fluid retention. This was accompanied by inhibition of sodium–potassium ATPase, leading to an increase in intracellular sodium and calcium that was thought to be responsible for the subsequent development of increased peripheral resistance and hypertension while plasma volume returned to normal. They did not, however, explain the mechanism by which the initial fluid retention occurred. Siamopoulos and Wilkinson[109] have found increased levels of plasma renin activity, plasma angiotensin II and plasma aldosterone in patients with chronic pyelonephritis and only mild renal impairment, suggesting that the fluid retention was probably renin dependent. The mechanism by which renin levels are elevated in response to renal damage is not established, but the rise may be a part of the adaptation to nephron loss that leads to hyperfiltration by remaining nephrons. Mansy et al.[110] have found an increase in plasma renin activity accompanying an increase in GFR and filtration fraction in normal subjects fed a high-protein diet, suggesting that efferent arteriolar constriction by angiotension II may be important in the hyperfiltration accompanying protein feeding and may also be important in the hyperfiltration by residual nephrons after nephron loss. The stimulation of aldosterone and subsequent fluid retention may also contribute to increased filtration through residual nephrons by raising systemic blood pressure and filtration pressure. Since some nephron loss is likely after initial acute tubular necrosis or acute rejection following transplantation, it seems likely that hypertension may result from a mechanism similar to that discussed above in relation to early renal disease.

•

References

1. Bachy, C., Alexandre, G. P. J. van Ypersele de Strihou, C. (1976). Hypertension after renal transplantation. *Br. Med. J.*, **2**, 1287–9
2. Rap, T. K. S., Gupta, S. K., Butt, K. H., Kountz, S. L. and Friedman, E. A. (1978). Relationship of renal transplantation to hypertension in end-stage renal failure. *Arch. Intern. Med.*, **138**, 1236–41
3. Wauthier, M., Vereerstraeten, P., Pirson, Y., Toussaint, C., Alexandre, G. P. J., Kinnaert, P., van Geertruyden, H. and van Ypersele de Strihou, C. (1982). Prevalence and causes of hypertension late after renal transplantation. *Proc. EDTA*, **19**, 566–71
4. Tejani, A. (1983). Post-transplant hypertension and hypertensive encephalopathy in renal allograft recipients. *Nephron*, **34**, 73–8
5. Najarian, J. S., Simmons, R. L., and Tallent, M. G. (1971). Renal transplantation in infants and children. *Ann. Surg.*, **174**, 583–93
6. Brunner, F. P., Brynger, H., Chantler, C., Donckerwolcke, R. A., Hathaway, R. A., Jacobs, C., Selwood, N. H. and Wing, A. J. (1979). Combined report on regular dialysis and transplantation in Europe. *Proc. EDTA*, **16**, 3–82
7. Registry Report. European Dialysis and Transplant Association Registry. Demography of dialysis and transplantation in Europe 1984. (1986). *Nephrol. Dial. Transplant.*, **1**, 1–8
8. Nicholls, A. J., Catto, G. D. R., Edward, N., Engeset, J. and MacLeod, M. (1980). Accelerated atherosclerosis in long-term dialysis and renal transplant patients: fact or fiction. *Lancet*, **1**, 276–8
9. Society for Actuaries. (1959). *Build and Blood Pressure Study*. (Chicago: Society for Actuaries)
10. MRC Working Party. (1985). MRC trial of treatment of mild hypertension: principal results. *Br. Med. J.*, **291**, 97–104
11. Horvath, J. S., Baxter, C., Furby, F., Hood, V., Johnson, J., McGrath, B. and Tiller, D. J. (1976). Plasma renin activity, plasma angiotensin II and extracellular fluid volume in patients after renal transplantation. *Clin. Sci. Mol. Med.*, **51**, 227s–30s
12. McHugh, M. I., Tanboga, H., Marcen, R., Liano, F., Robson, V. and Wilkinson, R. (1980). Hypertension following renal transplantation. The role of the host's kidneys. *Q. J. Med.*, **49**, 395–403
13. Popovtzer, M. M., Pinnggera, W., Katz, F. H., Corman, J. L., Robinette, J. Lanois, B., Halgrimson, C. G. and Starzl, T. E. (1973). Variations in arterial blood pressure after kidney transplantation. *Circulation*, **47**, 1297–1305
14. Snow, M. H., Jachuck, S. J., Robson, V. and Wilkinson, R. (1978). Plasma renin activity following renal transplantation. *Postgrad. Med. J.*, **54**, 311–7
15. Kornerup, H. J. and Pedersen, E. B. (1977). Plasma renin, plasma aldosterone and exchangeable sodium in normotensive and hypertensive kidney transplant recipients with and without transplant artery stenosis. *Acta Med. Scand.*, **202**, 509–16
16. Huysmans, F. T. M., Hoitsma, A. J. and Koene, R. A. P. (1986). Factors determining hypertension after renal transplantation. *Nephrol. Dial. Transplant*, **2**, 135
17. Jacquot, C., Idatte, J. M., Bedrossian, J., Weiss, Y., Safar, M. and Bariety, J.

(1978). Long-term blood pressure changes in renal homo-transplantation. *Arch. Intern. Med.*, **138**, 233–6

18. Cohen, S. L. (1973). Hypertension in renal transplant recipients: Role of bilateral nephrectomy. *Br. Med. J.*, **3**, 78–81
19. Pollini, J., Gittmann, R. D., Beaudoin, J. G., Morehouse, D. D., Kiassen, J. and Knaack, J. (1979). Late hypertension following renal allotransplantation. *Clin. Nephrol.*, **11**, 202–12
20. Turner, B. I., Richie, R. E., Johnson, K., MacDonell, R. C., Tallent, M. B. and Niblack, G. D. (1983). Bilateral nephrectomy concomitantly with renal transplantation. *J. Urol.*, **130**, 240–2
21. Coles, G. A., Crosby, D. L., Jones, G. R., Jones, J. H., and McVeigh, S. (1972). Hypertension following cadaveric renal transplantation. *Postgrad. Med. J.*, **48**, 399–404
22. Grollman, A. and Krishnamurty, V. S. R. (1971). A new pressor agent of renal origin: its differentiation from renin and angiotensin. *Am. J. Physiol.*, **221**, 1499–1503
23. Wilkinson, R., Scott, D. F., Uldall, P. R., Kerr, D. N. S., Swinney, J. and Robson, V. (1970). Plasma renin and exchangeable sodium in the hypertension of chronic renal failure. The effect of bilateral nephrectomy. *Q. J. Med.*, **39**, 377–94
24. Yarimizu, S. N., Susan, L. P., Straffon, R. A., Stewart, B. H., Magnusson, M. O. and Nakamoto, S. S. (1978). Mortality and morbidity in pretransplant bilateral nephrectomy. *Urology*, **12**, 55–8
25. Winearls, C. G., Oliver, D. O., Pippard, M. J., Reid, C., Downing, M. R. and Cotes, P. M. (1986). Effect of human erythropoietin derived from recombinant DNA on the anaemia of patients maintained by chronic haemodialysis. *Lancet*, **2**, 1175–8
26. Rai, G. S., Wilkinson, R., Taylor, R. M. R., Uldall,.P. R. and Kerr, D. N. S. (1978). Adverse effect of splenectomy in renal transplantation. *Clin. Nephrol.*, **9**, 194–9
27. Curtis, J. J. (1984). Hypertension after renal transplantation. *Alabama J. Med. Sci.*, **21**, 412–5
28. Ladefoged, J., Nerstrom, B. and Nielsen, I. (1974). The possible significance of renin determinations in selection of kidney-transplanted patients for bilateral nephrectomy in treatment of hypertension. *Scand. J. Urol. Nephrol.*, **8**, 240–1
29. Fyhrquist, F., Kock, B., Edgren, J., Wallenius, M., Kuhlbäck, B., Lindfors, O. and Lindström, B. (1975). Selective renin determinations in hypertensive renal transplant recipients. *N. Engl. J. Med.*, **293**, 1105
30. Khoury, G. A., Farrington, K., Varghese, Z., Persaud, J. W., Irving, J. D., Fernando, O. N., Moorhead, J. F. and Sweny, P. (1983). Digital vascular imaging and selective renin sampling in post-transplant hypertension. Which kidney is responsible? *Clin. Nephrol.*, **20**, 225–30
31. van Ypersele de Strihou, C., Vereerstraeten, P., Wauthier, M., Toussaint, C., Pirson, Y., de Plaen, J. F., Vanheerweghem, J. L., Dautrebande, J., Kinnaert, P., van Geertruyden, J., Dupont, E. and Alexandre, G. P. J. (1983). Prevalence, etiology and treatment of late post-transplant hypertension. *Advances in Nephrology 1983*. (Chicago: Year Book Medical Publishers, Inc.)
32. Grunfeld, J. P., Kleinknecht, D., Moreau, J. F., Kamoun, P., Sabto, J., Garcia-Torres, R., Osorio, M. and Kreis, H. (1975). Permanent hypertension after renal homotransplantation in man. *Clin. Sci.*, **48**, 391–403

33. Thompson, J. F., Fletcher, E. W. L., Wood, R. F. M., Chalmers, D. H. K., Taylor, H. M., Benjamin, I. S. and Morris, P. J. (1984). Control of hypertension after renal transplantation by embolisation of host kidneys. *Lancet*, **2**, 424–7

34. Huysmans, F. T. M., Hoitsma, A. J., Wetzels, J. F. M. and Koene, R.A.P. (1985). Blood pressure changes after embolisation of host kidney in renal transplant patients. *Lancet*, **1**, 344

35. Keller, F. S., Coyle, M., Rosch, J. and Dotter, C. T. (1986). Percutaneous renal ablation in patients with end-stage renal disease: alternative to surgical nephrectomy. *Radiology*, **159**, 447–51

36. Bianchi, G., Fox, U., DiFrancesco, G. F., Bardi, U. and Radice, M. (1973). The hypertensive role of the kidney in spontaneously hypertensive rats. *Clin. Sci. Mol. Med.*, **45**, 135s–9s

37. Curtis, J. J., Luke, R. G., Dustan, H. P., Kashgarian, M., Whelchel, J. D., Jones, P., and Diethelm, A. G. (1983). Remission of essential hypertension after renal transplantation. *N. Engl. J. Med.*, **309**, 1009–15

38. Guidi, E., Boanchi, V., Dallosta, V., Cantaluppi, A., Mandelli, V., Vallino, F. and Polli, E. (1982). Influence of familial hypertension of the donor on the blood pressure and antihypertensive therapy of kidney graft recipients. *Nephron*, **30**, 318–23

39. Guidi, E., Bianchi, G. Rivolta, E., Ponticelli, C., diPalo, F. Q., Minetti, L. and Pollo, E. (1985). Hypertension in man with a kidney transplant: role of familial versus other factors. *Nephron*, **41**, 14–21

40. Strandgaard, S. and Hansen, U. (1986). Hypertension in renal allograft recipients may be conveyed by cadaveric kidneys from donors with subarachnoid haemorrhage. *Br. Med. J.*, **292**, 1041

41. Faenza, A., Spolaore, R., Poggioli, G., Selleri, S., Roversi, R. and Gozzetti, G. (1983). Renal artery stenosis after renal transplantation. *Kidney Int.*, **23**, S54–S59

42. Nilson, A. E., Hendriksson, C. and Thoren, A. (1976). Angiographic diagnosis and follow up of artery stenosis in renal transplantation. *Scand. J. Urol. Nephrol.*, **Suppl 38**, 131

43. Jachuck, S. J., Wilkinson, R., Uldall, P. R., Elliott, R. W., Taylor, R. M. R., and Hacking, P. M. (1979). The medical management of renal artery stenosis in transplant recipients. *Br. J. Surg.*, **66**, 19–22

44. Whelton, P. K., Russell, R. P., Harrington, D. P., Williams, G. M. and Walker, W. G. (1979). Hypertension following renal transplantation. *J. Am. Med. Assoc.* **241**, 1128–31

45. Tilney, N. L., Rocha, A., Strom, T. B. and Kirkman, R. L. (1984). Renal artery stenosis in transplant patients. *Ann. Surg.*, **199**, 454–60

46. Dickerman, R. M., Peters, P. C., Hull, A. R., Curry, T. S., Atkins, C. and Fry, W. J. (1980). Surgical correction of post-transplant renovascular hypertension. *Ann. Surg.*, **192**, 639–44

47. Nghiem, D. D., Schulak, J. A., Bonsib, S. M., Ercolani, L. and Corry, R. J. (1984). Fibromuscular dysplasia: an unusual cause of hypertension in the transplant recipient. *Transplant Proc.*, **16**, 555–8

48. Ricotta, J. J., Schaff, H. V., Williamson, G. M., Rolley, R. T., Whelton, P. K. and Harrington, D. M. (1978). Renal artery stenosis following transplantation. Etiology, diagnosis and prevention. *Surgery*, **84**, 595–602

49. Jachuck, S. J. and Wilkinson, R. (1972) Abdominal bruit after renal transplantation. *Br. Med. J.*, **3**, 202–3
50. Anderson, C. F., Woods, J. E., Frohnert, P. P., Donadio, J. U., Suros, J., Sung, P. T. and Johnson W. J. (1973). Renal allograft bruit: an encouraging finding. *Mayo Clin. Proc.*, **48**, 13–7
51. Flechner, S. M., Sandler, C. M., Childs, T., Ben-Menachem, Y., van Buren, C. V., Payne, W. and Kahan, B. D. (1983). Screening for transplant renal artery stenosis in hypertensive recipients using digital subtraction angiography. *J. Urol.*, **130**, 339–43
52. Clark, R. A. and Alexander, E. S. (1983). Digital subtraction angiography of the renal arteries. Prospective comparison with conventional angiography. *Invest. Radiol.*, **18**, 6–8
53. Malfi, B., Triolo, G., Squiccimarro, G., Messina, M., Rossetti, M., Colla, L., Ferretti, G., Salomone, A., Segoloni, G. P. and Vercellone, A. (1986). Usefulness of echo-doppler velocimetry in the diagnosis of renal artery stenosis of the transplanted kidney. *Nephrol. Dial. Transplant*, **1**, 136
54. Sellars, L., Shore, A. C. and Wilkinson, R. (1985). Renal vein renin studies in renovascular hypertension – do they really help? *J. Hypertension*, **3**, 177–81
55. Curtis, J. J., Luke, R. G., Whelchel, J. D., Diethelm, A. G., Jones, P., and Dustan, H. P. (1983). Inhibition of angiotensin-converting enzyme in renal transplant recipients with hypertension. *N. Engl. J. Med.*, **308**, 377–81
56. Farrow, P. R. and Wilkinson, R. (1979). Reversible renal failure during treatment with Captopril. *Br. Med. J.*, **1**, 1680
57. Hricik, D. E., Browning, P. J., Kopelman, R., Goorno, W. E., Madias, N. E. and Dzau, V. J. (1983). Captopril-induced functional renal insufficiency in patients with bilateral renal artery stenosis or renal artery stenosis in a solitary kidney. *N. Engl. J. Med.*, **308**, 373–6
58. van der Woude, F. J., van Son, W. J., Tegzess, A. M., Donker, A. J. M., Slooff, M. J. H., van der Slikke, L. B. and Hoorntje, S. J. (1985). Effect of captopril on blood pressure and renal function in patients with transplant renal artery stenosis. *Nephron*, **39**, 184–8
59. Trachtman, H., Butt, K. M. H., Gordon, D. and Tejani, A. (1985). The use of captopril to control hypertension in post-transplant renal artery stenosis. *Clin. Nephrol.*, **23**, 203–6
60. Venkatachalam, K. and Kosanovich, J. M. (1983). Captopril in hypertension after renal transplantation. *Clin. Nephrol.*, **19**, 265–8
61. Luke, R. G., Curtis, J. J., Jones, P., Whelchel, J. D. and Diethelm, A. G. (1985). Mechanisms of post-transplant hypertension. *Am. J. Kidney Dis.*, **5**, A79–84
62. Dautrebande, J. Pirson, Y., van Ypersele de Strihou, C., Alexandre, G. P. and van Cangh, P. J. (1979). Reversible renal artery stenosis in renal transplantation. *Urology*, **13**, 529–31
63. Steensma-Vegter, A. J., Krediet, R. T., Westra, D. and Tegzess, A. M. (1981). Reversible stenosis of the renal artery in cadaver kidney grafts: a report of three cases. *Clin. Nephrol.*, **15**, 102–6
64. Chan, Y. T., Ng, W. D., Ho. C. P. and Lau, W. C. (1985). Reversible stenosis of the renal artery following renal transplantation. *Br. J. Surg.*, **72**, 454–5
65. Sagalowsky, A. I. and Peters, P. C. (1984). Renovascular hypertension following renal transplantation. *Urol. Clin. North Am.*, **11**, 491–502

66. Lohr, J. W., MacDougall, M. L., Chonko, A. M., Diederich, D. A., Grantham, J. J., Savin, V. J. and Wiegmann, T. B. (1986). Percutaneous transluminal angioplasty in transplant renal artery stenosis. Experience and review of the literature. *Am. J. Kidney Dis.*, **7**, 363–7

67. Chandrasoma, P. and Aberele, A. M. (1986). Anastomotic line renal artery stenosis after transplantation. *J. Urol.*, **135**, 1159–62

68. Baumgartner, D., Keusch, G., Retsch, M. and Largiader, F. (1984). Correction of renal transplant artery stenosis: Early and long-term results. *Transplant Proc.*, **16**, 1308–10

69. van Son, W. J., van der Woude, F. J., Tegzess, A. M., Donker, A. J. M., Slooff, M. J. H., van Slikke, B. and Hoorntje, S. J. (1983). Captopril induced deterioration of graft function in patients with a transplant renal artery stenosis. *Proc. EDTA*, **20**, 325–30

70. Sniderman, K. W., Sprayregen, S., Sos, T. A., Saddekni, S., Hilton, S., Mollenkopf, F. Soberman, R., Cheigh, J. S., Tapia, L., Stubenford, W., Tellis, V. and Veith, F. J. (1980). Percutaneous transluminal dilation in renal transplant arterial stenosis. *Transplantation*, **30**, 440–4

71. Campieri, C., Mignani, R., Feletti, C., Vangelista, A. and Bonomini, V. (1983). Percutaneous transluminal dilatation of post-transplant renal artery stenosis. Beneficial effects in two cases at high surgical risk. *Clin. Exp. Hyper. Theor. Prac.*, **A5**, 803–13

72. Campieri, C. and Bonomini, V. (1985). Percutaneous transluminal dilatation of graft renal artery stenosis as treatment for post-transplant hypertension. *Nephron*, **40**, 120–1

73. Mollenkopf, F. P., Matas, A. J. and Veith, F. J. (1982). Percutaneous transluminal angioplasty for transplant renal artery stenosis. Presented at the *Ninth International Congress Transplant Society, Brighton, 1982.* Quoted in reference 65 (q.v.)

74. Majeski, J. A. and Munda, R. (1981). Hazard of percutaneous transluminal dilation in renal transplant arterial stenosis. *Arch. Surg.*, **116**, 1225–6

75. Legrain, M., Michon, F., Cluckman, J. C., Beaufils, H. and Kuss, R. (1973). Arterial hypertension during the first three months following renal transplantation. *J. d'Urologie et de Néphrologie*, **79**, 444–450

76. Friedman, E. A., Chou, L. M., Beyer, M. M., Butt, K. M. H. and Manis, T. (1985). Adverse impact of hypertension on diabetic recipients of transplanted kidneys. *Hypertension*, 7 (Suppl. II), 131–4

77. Anderson, S., Meyer, T. W. and Brenner, B. M. (1985). The role of hemodynamic factors in the initiation and progression of renal disease. *J. Urol.*, **133**, 363–8

78. Hall, J. E., Morse, C. L., Smith, M. J., Young, D. B. and Guyton, A. C. (1980). Control of arterial pressure and renal function during glucocorticoid excess in dogs. *Hypertension*, **2**, 139–48

79. McHugh, M. I., Tanboga, H. and Wilkinson, R. (1980). Alternate day steroids and blood pressure control after renal transplantation. *Proc. EDTA*, **17**, 496–501

80. Sampson, D. and Albert, D. J. (1973). Alternate day therapy with methylprednisolone after renal transplantation. *J. Urol.*, **109**, 345–52

81. Ingelfinger, J. R. (1981). *Hypertension in Children with Kidney Transplants.* (Boston: Nijhoff)

82. Tuck, M. L., Sowers, J., Dornfeld, L., Kledzik, G. and Maxwell, M. (1981). The effect of weight reduction on blood pressure, plasma renin activity, and plasma aldosterone levels in obese patients. *N. Engl. J. Med.*, **304**, 930–3

83. Swales, J. D. (1980). Dietary salt and hypertension. *Lancet*, **1**, 1177–9

84. MacGregor, G. A., Markandu, N. D., Best, F. E., Elder, D. M., Cam, J. M., Sagnella, G. A. and Squires, M. (1982). Double blind randomised crossover trial of moderate sodium restriction in essential hypertension. *Lancet*, **1**, 351–5

85. Kalbfleisch, J. H., Hebert, L. A., Lemann, J., Piering, W. F. and Beres, J. A. (1982). Habitual excessive dietary salt intake and blood pressure levels in renal transplant recipients. *Am. J. Med.*, **73**, 205–10

86. Curtis, J. J., Luke, R. G., Jones, P., Diethelm, A. G. and Whelchel, J. D. (1985). Hypertension after successful renal transplantation. *Am. J. Med.*, **79**, 193–200

87. The Canadian Transplant Study Group (1985). Examination of parameters influencing the benefit:detriment ratio of cyclosporin in renal transplantation. *Am. J. Kidney Dis.*, **5**, 328–32

88. Henny, G. C., Kootte, A. M. M., van Beckel, J. H., Baldwin, W. M., Hermans, J., Bos, B., van Es, L. A. and Paul, L. C. (1986). A prospective randomised comparative study on the influence of cyclosporin and azathioprine on renal allograft survival and function. *Nephrol. Dial. Transplant.*, **1**, 44–9

89. Ferguson, R. M., Rynasiewicz, J. J., Sutherland, D. E., Simmons, R. L. and Najarian, J. S. (1982). Cyclosporin A in renal transplantation: a prospective randomised trial. *Surgery*, **92**, 175–82

90. Loughran, T. P., Deeg, H. J., Dahlberg, S., Kennedy, M. S. Storb, R. and Thomas, E. D. (1985). Incidence of hypertension after marrow transplantation among 112 patients randomised to either cyclosporin or methotrexate as graft versus host disease prophylaxis. *Br. J. Haematol.*, **59**, 547–53

91. Chapman, J. R. and Morris, P. J. (1985). Cyclosporin nephrotoxicity and the consequences of conversion to azathioprine. *Transplant Proc.*, **17**, (Suppl. 1), 254–60

92. Curtis, J. J., Dubosky, E., Whelchel, J. D., Luke, R. G., Diethelm A. G. and Hones, P. (1986). Cyclosporin in therapeutic doses increases renal allograft vascular resistance. *Lancet*, **2**, 477–9

93. Deray, G., LeHoang, P., Achour, L., Hornych, A., Landault, C. and Caraillon, A. (1986). Cyclosporin and Raynaud phenomenon. *Lancet*, **2**, 1092–3

94. Myers, B. D., Ross, J., Newton, L., Leutscher, J. A. and Perlroth, M. (1984). Cyclosporin-associated chronic nephropathy. *N. Engl. J. Med.*, **311**, 699–705

95. Zinman, L. and Libertino, J. A. (1982) Uncommon disorders of the renal circulation. In Breslin, D. J., Swinton, N. W., Libertino, J. A. and Zinman, L. (eds.) *Renovascular Hypertension*, pp. 118–20. (Baltimore: Williams & Wilkins)

96. Smith, R. S., Albano, J., Reid, J. L. and Warren, D. J. (1983). Increased vascular sensitivity to noradrenaline in hypertensive renal transplant recipients. *Transplantation*, **36**, 666–70

97. Kim, K. E., Bates, O., Lyons, P., Pitone, J., Martinez, E. W., Valvo, E., Sabanayagam, P., Bower, R., Swartz, C. and Onesti, G. (1980). Haemodynamics of stable renal transplant recipients. *Clin. Sci.*, **59**, 377s–9s

98. Sampson, D., Kirdani, R. Y., Sandberg, A. A. and Murphy, G. P. (1972). The renin aldosterone relationship after renal allotransplantation in man. *Invest. Urol.*, **10**, 66–8

99. Baumann, K., Nussberger, J., Schmied, U., Vetter, W., Zaruba, K., Largiader, F. and Binswanger, U. (1975). Plasma renin activity and plasma aldosterone in hypertensive kidney allograft recipients. *Proc. EDTA*, **12**, 471–6

100. Linas, S. L., Miller, P. D., McDonald, K. M., Stables, D. P., Katz, F., Weil, R. and Schrier, R. W. (1978). Role of the renal angiotensin system in post-transplantation hypertension in patients with multiple kidneys. *N. Engl. J. Med.*, **298**, 1440–4

101. Bennett, W. M., McDonald, W. J., Lawson, R. K., and Porter, G. A. (1974). Post transplant hypertension: Studies of cortical blood flow and the renal pressor system. *Kidney Int.*, **6**, 99–108

102. Curtis, J. J., Luke, R. G., Whelchel, J. D. *et al.* (1984). Role of native kidneys in post-transplant hypertension. *Kidney Int.*, **24**, 341

103. Coleman, T. G. and Guyton, A. C. (1969). Hypertension caused by salt loading in the dog. Onset transients of cardiac output and other circulatory variables. *Circ. Res.*, **25**, 152–60

104. de Wardener, H. E. and MacGregor, G. A. (1980). Dahl's hypothesis that a saluretic substance may be responsible for a sustained rise in arterial pressure: its possible role in essential hypertension. *Kidney Int.*, **18**, 1–9

105. Brown, T. C., Davis, J. O., Olichney, M. J. and Johnston, C. I. (1966). Relation of plasma renin to sodium balance and arterial pressure in experimental renal hypertension. *Circ. Res.*, **18**, 475–83

106. Tobian, L., Coffee, K. and McCrea, P. (1969). Contrasting exchangeable sodium in rats with different types of Goldblatt hypertension. *Am. J. Physiol.*, **217**, 458–60

107. Brod, J., Bahlmann, J., Cachovan, M. and Pretschner, P. (1983). Development of hypertension in renal disease. *Clin. Sci.*, **64**, 141–52

108. Brod, J., Schaeffer, J., Hengstenberg, J. H. and Kleinschmidt, T. H. (1984). Investigations on the sodium potassium pump in erythrocytes of patients with renal hypertension. *Clin. Sci.*, **66**, 351–5

109. Siamopoulos, K. and Wilkinson, R. (1987). Hypertension in chronic pyelo-nephritis. *Contr. Nephrol.*, **54**, 119–23

110. Mansy, H., Patel, D., Tapson, J. S., Fernandez, J., Tapster, S., Torrance, A. D. and Wilkinson, R. (1987). Four methods to recruit renal functional reserve. *Nephrol., Dial. Transplant.*, **2**, 228–32

6

HYPERTENSION IN PREGNANCY

D. RUSSO, A. DAL CANTON and V. E. ANDREUCCI

Hypertension in pregnancy remains a major cause of maternal and fetal morbidity and mortality[1]. Hypertension may either precede pregnancy ('chronic hypertension in pregnancy') or occur in a previously normotensive woman from a disorder of pregnancy itself ('pregnancy-induced hypertension').

PREGNANCY-INDUCED HYPERTENSION (PIH)

Pregnancy-induced hypertension usually occurs after 24 weeks of gestation (rarely before 20 weeks). It may occur alone or, more often, in association with proteinuria and/or oedema. When this association is present, the syndrome is also called 'toxaemia of pregnancy', 'pre-eclampsia', or 'EPH gestosis' (E, oedema, P. proteinuria; H, hypertension). Preeclampsia is predominantly a disease of nulliparous women, occurring most commonly at the extremes of reproductive age (teenagers or women over 35 years). It may occur in multiparae with any of the following conditions: multifetal pregnancy, fetal hydrops, hydatiform mole, Rh incompatibility, maternal vascular diseases such as hypertensive nephropathies, essential hypertension, diabetes mellitus, or autoimmune disorders with vascular damage such as systemic lupus erythematosus or scleroderma[2,3]. PIH may lead to 'eclampsia', which is characterized by preeclampsia plus convulsions resulting from pregnancy-induced hypertension.

The diagnosis of PIH may be made when blood pressure is 140/90 or greater or when there has been an increase of 30 mmHg in systolic blood pressure or 15 mmHg in diastolic blood pressure over the pre-pregnancy values on at least two occasions 6 hours or more apart[3]. The severity of PIH is indicated not only by a high blood pressure (diastolic blood pressure of 110 mmHg or higher) but also by the association of proteinuria, headache, visual disturbances, epigastric or right upper quadrant abdominal pain (presumably due to hepatic oedema and subcapsular haemorrhage), oliguria, convulsions, thrombocytopenia, hyperbilirubinaemia, increases in serum creatinine levels and SGOT and obvious fetal growth retardation. It should be stressed that blood pressure alone is not always indicative of severity; thus, convulsions may occur in a patient with diastolic blood pressure of 90 mmHg but not in a patient with 120 mmHg. Furthermore, mild PIH may suddenly become severe. Whatever the blood pressure, convulsions indicate the onset of eclampsia. The seizures of eclampsia are similar to those of *grand mal* epilepsy and may appear before or during labour, or even postpartum (within 48 hours – after this time it is more likely that seizures are the consequence of other lesions of the central nervous system)[3].

Pathogenesis of pregnancy-induced hypertension

The pathogenetic mechanism of PIH is still obscure. Many theories have been proposed. The demonstration that antisera to trophoblastic tissue cross-react with renal tissue, the observation of immunoglobulins and complement in renal lesions of patients with PIH, and the detection of circulating immune complexes in preeclampsia have raised the possibility of an immunological mechanism[4-8]. This seems to be supported by the observation[9] of a much greater incidence of preeclampsia in primiparae (25.4%) than in multiparae (9.6%), suggesting that the first pregnancy confers protection against preeclampsia[9], even when the first pregnancy ended in abortion[9,10]; the incidence of PIH in the second pregnancy after an abortion was significantly lower than in a first pregnancy, but higher than in multiparae, suggesting only partial protection by abortion[9]. A recent study, however, has proposed different pathophysiological mechanisms in primiparous and multiparous pregnant women with PIH,

194

despite similar clinical presentations[11]. In this study, in comparison with hypertensive primiparae, hypertensive multiparae exhibited (a) an earlier increase in arterial pressure, (b) a longer time between the first rise in blood pressure and delivery, and (c) lower maternal weight gain. Furthermore, neonates born to hypertensive multiparae exhibited a lower birth weight increase with parity when compared with babies from control (non-hypertensive) multiparous women – this phenomenon, usually associated with growth-retarded, calcified and insufficient placentas, suggests a diminished nutritional support to the fetus during multiparous hypertensive pregnancy[11]. These observations appear to indicate a clear difference in pathogenetic mechanisms, rather than two expressions of the same mechanism in PIH.

Disseminated intravascular coagulation has also been implicated in the pathogenesis of PIH[12,13].

Uteroplacental ischaemia is widely recognized as a primary event. On the basis of recent studies, the following hypothesis has been suggested for preeclampsia[2]. Two main organs are involved in preeclampsia: uterus and kidney. Both are producers of renin and prostaglandins. Normal pregnant women are refractory to the pressor effects of angiotensin II[14]. This refractoriness appears to be mediated by vascular tissue synthesis of a prostaglandin, prostacyclin (PGI2) or prostaglandin E2 (PGE2) or a prostaglandin-like substance, and is abolished by aspirin or indomethacin (prostaglandin synthetase inhibitors)[15]. Preeclampsia is characterized by increased vascular sensitivity to angiotensin II and other vasoconstrictor agents. This may be caused by a deficiency in PGI2 production, since PGI2 generation in fetal and maternal blood vessels has been shown to be reduced in preeclampsia[2,16-21]. PIH is also associated with increased production of thromboxane A2 (a potent vasoconstrictor and stimulator of platelet aggregation) by the placenta[22] and by platelets[23]. Hence, thromboxane A2 may contribute to the vasoconstriction, platelet hyperactivity and uteroplacental thrombosis of preeclampsia; these phenomena are prevented by aspirin[24]. Gant et al.[3,25] have demonstrated that the increased vascular sensitivity to angiotensin II precedes the occurrence of preeclampsia, thereby causing the generalized vasoconstriction and increase in systemic blood pressure. The resulting severe reduction in uteroplacental blood flow (by approximately 50%)[26] will cause uteroplacental ischaemia and increase the uteroplacental production not only of renin but also consequently, of angiotensin II. This will lead to a greater generalized vasoconstriction (including the uteroplacental vasculature) and PIH[2,3]. Thus, the loss of vascular refractoriness to angiotensin II, presumably due to a PGI2 deficiency, seems to play a central role in the pathogenesis of preeclampsia.

Clinical aspects of pregnancy-induced hypertension

The two important signs of PIH, i.e. hypertension and proteinuria, are usually asymptomatic and the pregnant woman is thus not usually aware of being ill. When symptoms such as headache, visual disturbances or abdominal pain occur, the disease is already severe. Hence there is need for adequate education of pregnant women to ensure that they have frequent blood pressure measurements throughout gestation, particularly in the second half, have monthly urinalyses, and seek medical advice for any unusual symptoms that may occur. Any increase in diastolic blood pressure to or above 90 mmHg is abnormal. The normal diurnal blood pressure rhythm may be reversed, with highest levels during the night and early in the morning; furthermore, the hypertension is often labile because of the increased sensitivity to vasopressor hormones[1]. A sudden increase in body weight, which is frequently the first sign of PIH, should also be regarded as abnormal. An increase in body weight of about 1 pound per week is normal; but an increase in body weight of more than 2 pounds in a week or 6 pounds in a month should suggest the possibility of preeclampsia; it is the rate of the excessive weight gain (rather than excessive gain distributed throughout gestation) that is the important sign[3]. This sudden excessive increase in body weight (in some cases it may reach 10 pounds or more in a week) is due to fluid retention. Usually the weight gain precedes visible signs of salt and water retention, such as swollen eyelids or puffiness of the fingers, oedema and oliguria[27].

Headache, usually frontal (sometimes occipital), is frequent in severe cases and precedes convulsions. The headache is often resistant to analgesics. Visual disturbances (from slight blurring of vision to blindness) are attributed to retinal vasospasm, ischaemia and oedema; in rare cases it is due to retinal detachment[3]. Retinal exudates and haemorrhages are very unusual in PIH; when present they indicate chronic hypertension preceding pregnancy.

Proteinuria usually occurs after hypertension and often shows considerable variation in quantity between individuals and within any individual from time to time. In some cases it may reach 10 grams per day but resolves after delivery.

Epigastric or right upper quadrant abdominal pain occurs only in severe preeclampsia and is presumably due to hepatic oedema and subcapsular haemorrhage, with consequent stretching of the hepatic capsule. This symptom is frequently followed by convulsions.

Prognosis of pregnancy-induced hypertension

PIH is an important complication of pregnancy and may not only result in maternal death but is one of the important causes of perinatal mortality and morbidity. Prognosis for mother and fetus is variable and depends on the gestional age of the fetus, whether the condition is adequately treated, when delivery occurs and whether eclampsia supervenes. Usually, blood pressure returns to normal within 2 weeks of delivery.

Whether preeclampsia causes chronic hypertension remains a matter of controversy. There are long-term follow-up studies that suggest that preeclampsia does not cause a greater incidence of hypertension later in life[28,29]. Other studies suggest that women who have had preeclampsia represent a risk group for future essential hypertension, since 30–40% of them will develop hypertension within 10–15 years[30,31]. The actual blood pressure level during pregnancy is less important than the blood pressure before or early in pregnancy[32,33]. According to recent studies, even children born after a hypertensive pregnancy seem to represent a risk group for future hypertension, since their blood pressure is higher than that of children born after normotensive pregnancy[34,35]. In our opinion, women who have had preeclampsia should be followed-up for many years.

Prevention of pregnancy-induced hypertension

Prevention is based on a thorough examination of the pregnant woman at frequent intervals throughout gestation, particularly of those who are predisposed to preeclampsia, and on early detection of the first signs (sudden weight gain, tendency of blood pressure to increase). In the last trimester of the pregnancy, women should be examined every two weeks and, in the last month, every week[3].

Diuretic drugs, such as thiazides, have been used in the past in an attempt to prevent the development of preeclampsia but were ineffective[36]. No benefit was observed with prophylactic hydrochlorothiazide[37]. In our opinion, the use of diuretics may be dangerous and may theoretically precipitate preeclampsia[38] through a reduction of renal and uteroplacental perfusion[39]. We believe that even dietary restriction of sodium intake in pregnant women should be avoided (see later).

Treatment of pregnancy-induced hypertension

When preeclampsia occurs in women at or near term, careful induction of labour and delivery is the best method of preserving both maternal health and fetal life.

With mild preeclampsia, bedrest throughout the day is very important. The patient may stay at home but must be examined twice weekly. When the patient is nulliparous, the diastolic blood pressure is greater than 90 mmHg (or systolic blood pressure is greater than 140 mmHg), and/or other symptoms are present, urinary (proteinuria) and blood tests (plasma creatinine, haematocrit, platelets, serum SGOT) should be performed; blood pressure should be measured every 4 hours and body weight should be checked every day.

Management includes control of blood pressure and prevention of seizures. Fortunately, in most cases, preeclampsia is mild and occurs sufficiently near to term that hypertension can be managed until labour commences spontaneously or can be safely induced[3]. When the fetus is premature, delivery should if possible be delayed; a few more weeks *in utero* reduces the risks of perinatal mortality and morbidity.

In severe preeclampsia (as in eclampsia), anticonvulsant (magnesium sulphate) and antihypertensive therapy become necessary, followed by delivery. Preeclampsia is cured by the expulsion of the trophoblast (i.e. by delivery). Delay in treating eclampsia or severe preeclampsia may be dangerous to the mother and fatal for the fetus. Since convulsions are more frequent during the period of labour and delivery, Gant *et al.*[3] suggest the use of intramuscular magnesium sulphate during labour and the early puerperium (24 hours post-partum) in all women suspected of having pregnancy-induced hyper-tension. Labour may be induced by oxytocin; should this induction be unsuccessful, a caesarean section is necessary[3].

After delivery there is almost invariably an immediate improvement; sometimes, however, there may be a transient worsening of the condition. Eclampsia may occur during labour or within 24 hours of delivery; hence the need for continuing therapy with magnesium sulphate and hydralazine for 24 hours postpartum[3]. Usually blood pressure returns to normal within 2 weeks of delivery.

Eclampsia

Clinical aspects of eclampsia

Eclampsia is an acute clinical condition characterized by tonic and clonic convulsions following pregnancy-induced hypertension. It occurs usually in the last trimester of pregnancy, becoming more frequent as term approaches. In addition to antepartum eclampsia, there may be intrapartum (during labour) and postpartum (within 24 hours after delivery) eclampsia. Apprehension, hyperexcitability and hyperreflexia frequently precede convulsions. In mild cases, there are only a few convulsions; in more severe cases, 10, 20 or up to 100 or more convulsions may occur. Sometimes, in untreated cases, the frequency is such that the patient convulses continuously[3].

The patient usually recovers consciousness after each eclamptic convulsion. Respiration is rapid (50 or more per minute). There is usually oliguria, proteinuria, oedema, and rarely haemoglobinuria and haemoglobinaemia. After delivery, an increase in urinary output indicates improvement; proteinuria and oedema disappear within a week, hypertension within two weeks[3].

Cyanosis and fever (39–40°C) are sometimes present and indicate a

199

grave prognosis. In severe cases, profound coma persists between convulsions and the patient dies without awakening, usually from a massive cerebral haemorrhage. Rarely, a sublethal haemorrhage causes hemiplegia, or eclampsia is followed by psychosis (lasting 1–2 weeks). On awakening from the coma, the patient may be blind because of retinal ischaemia, oedema, or, rarely, retinal detachment. Blindness usually disappears within a week[3].

Antepartum eclampsia usually accelerates labour; intrapartum eclampsia shortens it. Less frequently, labour does not commence, eclampsia is reversed, and pregnancy continues normally; in these cases a second and more severe episode of eclampsia may occur after a few days of preeclampsia. Pulmonary oedema, cyanosis and hypotension may appear terminally[3].

Treatment of eclampsia

As mentioned, eclampsia is cured with delivery. Hence, the treatment should consist in controlling convulsions and accelerating labour once the patient is free of convulsions and possibly conscious.

Gant et al.[3] suggest the following treatment for convulsions. Four grams of magnesium sulphate (20% solution) should be given intravenously, at a rate of 1 g/min followed by 10 g of 50% solution of magnesium sulphate i.m. (5 g deeply in each buttock; 1 ml of 2% Lidocaine (lignocaine) may be added to minimize discomfort). After 15 minutes, should convulsions persist, another 2 g of magnesium sulphate may be given intravenously (1 g/min). Then, every 4 hours, 5 g of a 50% of magnesium sulphate should be injected deeply i.m. in alternate buttocks provided that (a) the patellar reflex is present, (b) there is no depression of respiration, and (c) urine output in the preceding four hours was at least 100 ml. Magnesium sulphate should be discontinued 24 hours after delivery. Only on the rare occasions when convulsions do not disappear with magnesium sulphate, sodium amobarbital (amylobarbitone) may be slowly injected intravenously, (up to 0.25 g in not less than 3 minutes). The same treatment may be used during the first postictal hour if the eclamptic woman has not regained complete consciousness and shows physical agitation that cannot be easily controlled by gentle restraint. Agitation can be minimized by maintaining darkness and silence in the room and few people at the bedside (only one member of the family should be allowed in the room)[3].

Magnesium sulphate has some transient antihypertensive effects. Should diastolic blood pressure persist at 110 mmHg or more, hydralazine is given at a dosage of 5 mg i.v., with blood pressure monitored every 5 minutes. Should diastolic blood pressure not decrease to 90–100 mmHg in 20 minutes, 10 mg hydralazine are given i.v. and the dose repeated every 20 minutes until a diastolic blood pressure of 90–100 mmHg is attained. Usually, 5–20 mg of hydralazine are sufficient; hydralazine should be given again if diastolic blood pressure rises to 110 mmHg[3].

Gant et al.[3] are against the use of diazoxide (a potent peripheral vasodilator), which may be dangerous for both mother (maternal deaths following profound hypotension have been reported) and fetus (perinatal mortality and fetal distress have been observed) and may impair or arrest labour (diazoxide is a uterine relaxant). It has recently been demonstrated, however, that diazoxide can be safely used in the form of mini-bolus injections of 30 mg every 1–2 minutes[40]. Thus, in 34 patients with blood pressure greater than 160/115 (8 of whom had preexisting mild essential hypertension) mini-bolus diazoxide (30 mg) was given intravenously for 30–60 seconds (in addition to magnesium sulphate as anticonvulsant therapy) and repeated every 1–2 minutes until a diastolic blood pressure of less than 90 mmHg was achieved; the average required dose was 120 mg, with a maximum of 150 mg. No maternal hypotension occurred and maternal side-effects were minimal; neither perinatal mortality nor fetal distress were observed[40].

Prognosis of eclampsia

Prognosis is serious for both mother and fetus. Maternal mortality has fallen in recent years, but still ranges between zero and 17.5%; perinatal mortality varies between 13% and 30%[3].

CHRONIC HYPERTENSION IN PREGNANCY (CHP)

Treatment during pregnancy of hypertension that was known to be present before conception is, with only a few exceptions, usually disregarded in books both for obstetricians and for nephrologists. On the other hand, diagnosis of chronic hypertension in pregnancy is sometimes difficult because blood pressure normally decreases during pregnancy, so that a hypertensive woman may appear normotensive during the first trimester; the subsequent occurrence of hypertension may be erroneously regarded as preeclampsia.

There is still controversy as to whether mild hypertension antedating pregnancy should be treated in pregnant women. Some authors are against treatment because, in their opinion, the possible benefits of restoring blood pressure to normal are not relevant – given the brief span of gestation[36]. Others emphasize that treatment of chronic hypertension in pregnancy reduces the occurrence of superimposed preeclampsia, abruption, acute renal failure (due to acute tubular necrosis or renal cortical necrosis), retardation of intrauterine growth and midtrimester abortion[41,42]. In our opinion, there are important indications for continous treatment of essential hypertension during pregnancy. (a) CHP, regardless of its cause, is a predisposing factor to the development of superimposed preeclampsia; there is evidence[43,44] that the greater the diastolic blood pressure, the higher the incidence of preeclampsia. (b) CHP may cause cardiac decompensation. (c) Placental abruption is more frequent in hypertensive pregnant women. In principle, therefore, blood pressure equal to or greater than 140/90 mmHg must be treated.

Effect of antihypertensive therapy on cerebral blood flow and placental blood flow

Treatment of hypertension may affect both cerebral and placental blood flow. Cerebral blood flow is autoregulated, since it remains constant with variations in mean arterial pressure (diastolic blood pressure plus one-third of difference between systolic and diastolic pressure) between 70 and 150 mmHg[45]. Above the upper limit and below the lower limit of this autoregulatory range, hypertensive encephalopathy and cerebral ischaemia, respectively, may occur[36]. The lower and upper limits of the autoregulatory range are higher than normal in patients with chronic hypertension[46]. Hence, chronic hypertensive patients are more tolerant of higher pressures but less tolerant of lower pressures than are normotensive subjects[36]. When treating hypertension in pregnant women, therefore, blood pressure should be reduced to values at which cerebral blood flow is autoregulated.

Placental blood flow is not autoregulated; thus, it depends only on arterial blood pressure[36]. The occurrence of maternal hypotension may cause fetal bradycardia because of hypoxaemia. Since placental blood flow is reduced in preeclampsia and a maternal syndrome similar to preeclampsia may be induced in experimental animals by reducing placental blood flow, excessive lowering of systemic blood pressure by antihypertensive therapy may induce preeclampsia[38].

Antihypertensive drugs (Table 6.1)

Unfortunately, not all the antihypertensive medications available today have been adequately evaluated in pregnant hypertensive

TABLE 6.1   Antihypertensive drugs in pregnancy

Drugs	Dosage
Diuretics	Use limited to emergencies
β-Blockers	
Propranolol	40–240 mg daily
Oxprenolol	80–640 mg daily
Metroprolol	50–225 mg daily
Acebutolol	200–800 mg daily
Atenolol	50–100 mg daily
Labetalol	300–1200 mg daily
Hydralazine	50–200 mg daily
Calcium antagonists	
Nifedipine	10–40 mg daily
Methyldopa	750 mg–4 g daily
Clonidine	750–1500 μg daily
Converting enzyme inhibitors	
Captopril	should not be used
Enalapril	should not be used
Ganglion-blocking agents	should not be used

women. Methyldopa and, unfortunately, diuretics are the most widely used antihypertensive drugs[47] but many reported studies make no distinction between pregnancy-induced hypertension and chronic hypertension in pregnancy.

Diuretics

Thiazides have been used in the past to prevent the development of preeclampsia but have not been shown to have prophylactic value[36,41]. No difference in the incidence of preeclampsia was observed when pregnant women were treated with either hydrochlorothiazide or placebo during the last 16 weeks of gestation[37].

Whether diurectics are deleterious to the mother, to the fetus, or both remain controversial. Some experts believe that diuretics may be given in pregnancy[36] while others[3,48] warn of increases both in complications during labour and in perinatal mortality[49]. Despite some recent reports that there is no significant difference in perinatal outcome between patients treated with diuretics and untreated patients[43], the use of diuretics in chronic hypertension in pregnancy may in our opinion be dangerous. Theoretically, diuretics may precipitate preeclampsia, since (a) blood volume is commonly reduced not only in pregnancy-induced hypertension, but also in chronic hypertension in pregnancy; (b) hypovolaemia seems to precede and probably initiates preeclampsia; (c) diuretic therapy itself causes a reduction in blood volume; and (d) a decrease both in creatinine clearance and in uteroplacental perfusion has been demonstrated following diuretic therapy[39,50]. It has been recently suggested that diurectics should be given in association with methyldopa, as the salt and water retention caused by methyldopa would offset the volume contraction caused by thiazides[43]. In our opinion, the use of diurectics in pregnancy should be limited to emergencies, e.g. for treating left ventricular failure[3,36,48,51].

We believe that even dietary restriction of sodium should be avoided in women with CHP in order to prevent volume depletion. In a large prospective study (including more than 2000 pregnant women) the incidence of preeclampsia was less in pregnant women on a high-salt diet than those on a low-salt diet[52].

β-Blockers

β-Blockers have been widely used in pregnancy for treating idiopathic hypertrophic subaortic stenosis, hyperthyroidism, tachydysrhythmias and hypertension[53]. Since uterine activity is under adrenergic control, β-adrenergic blockade might theoretically enhance uterine activity and cause premature labour[54]. β-Blocking drugs have been used for many years[55] and this potential effect has not been mentioned in a recent important review[36,53].

Propranolol

There are only a few prospective studies on the use of propranolol in the treatment of essential hypertension in pregnancy. Eight out of nine pregnancies ended without problems for the severely hypertensive mothers and for their children after treatment with propranolol (up to 240 mg daily) plus hydralazine and a diuretic during pregnancy[56].

Good results have also been obtained in women in whom previous pregnancies have proved unsuccessful (abortions or stillbirths). In 25 hypertensive women who had experienced 67 pregnancies, 32 of which (47.8%) had been unsuccessful, treatment of hypertension with propranolol (40–160 mg daily) throughout the subsequent pregnancies reduced the incidence of unsuccessful pregnancies to 4 out of 26 (15.4%)[57]. Similarly, in 13 hypertensive women, who had previously experienced 17 unsuccessful pregnancies out of 38 (44.8%), treatment with propranolol (30–240 mg daily) plus hydralazine throughout the subsequent 15 pregnancies resulted in only one unsuccessful pregnancy (6.7%), which ended in a stillbirth[58].

It has been stated that treatment of pregnant women with propranolol is followed by respiratory distress in the neonate, increased perinatal mortality, and neonatal bradycardia or hypoglycaemia; but this statement is based on anecdotal reports and on retrospective study by chart review in which no information is given concerning other risk factors[59]. Thus, in a recent report, 3 out of 5 pregnant women treated with propranolol had stillbirths; but the β-blocker was given along with methyldopa and a thiazide because of the severity of the hypertension. The authors themselves suggest that the poor results with propranolol were probably due to the severity of hypertension rather than to the use of the drug[43].

205

Propranolol seems to be safe. It is commonly used in pregnancy at a dosage of 40–240 mg per day[1]. No fetal malformations have been reported, even when therapy was started before conception[56,58]. No intrauterine fetal growth retardation has been reported, and transient neonatal bradycardia or hypoglycaemia has been observed only occasionally in the few prospective studies of propranolol in which neonatal data are available[53,56,58].

Oxprenolol

There are only two randomized controlled trials in the literature on the use of oxprenolol (which was compared with methyldopa) in treating hypertension in pregnant women. In one of these studies[60] 50 patients were treated with oxprenolol (maximum daily dose, 640 mg) and 50 with methyldopa (maximum daily dose, 3 g); hydralazine had to be added to reduce diastolic blood pressure to less than 95 mmHg to six patients in the oxprenolol group and two patients in the methyldopa group. The results did not show any significant difference in the outcome of pregnancy between the two groups. Birth weight, placental weight and head circumference were not significantly different; there were no stillbirths in either group[60].

In the other randomized study[61], on 183 hypertensive pregnant women, 96 patients were treated with oxprenolol (80 mg to 640 mg daily) and 87 with methyldopa (500 mg up to 3 g daily). In 64 patients hydralazine (25 mg up to 300 mg daily) was also necessary to obtain a diastolic blood pressure lower than 85 mmHg. There were four perinatal deaths in the methyldopa group and one in the oxprenolol group. In contrast to the other study[60], fetal growth was greater in the oxprenolol group, probably due to peripheral vasodilatation induced by the drug. No neonatal hypoglycaemia was observed. Urgent delivery because of the severity of the condition was required for 10 patients in each group, all of whom exhibited proteinuria; this incidence of proteinuria is much lower than that reported in untreated hypertensive pregnant patients, suggesting a protective effect of therapy with β-blockers on superimposed preeclampsia. The authors of this study advocated the use of oxprenolol rather than methyldopa in the treatment of hypertensive pregnant women, provided that there is no contraindication to the administration of β-blockers[61].

Metoprolol

Theoretically, β-1-selective adrenoceptor blocking agents should be preferred in treating hypertensive pregnant women[62], because pregnancy is associated with a hyperkinetic circulation due to high sympathetic activity[63] and these drugs would have less effect on the uterine activity than unselective β-blockers[62]. Metoprolol is used in pregnancy at a dosage of 50–225 mg per day[1].

In a prospective study of the effect of metoprolol on 198 hypertensive pregnant women (about one-third of whom had preeclampsia) who were unresponsive to thiazides[64] the patients were divided in two groups. In one group of 101 patients, metoprolol was given either alone or (in 44 patients) associated with hydralazine; in the second group of 97 patients, hydralazine alone was given at a dosage up to 200 mg daily. The patients in both groups continued the thiazide throughout the study. There were 13 fetal or perinatal deaths in the hydralazine group and only three in the metoprolol group; no distinction was made between pregnancy-induced hypertension and essential hypertension[64].

In another randomized controlled trial, 161 hypertensive pregnant women were either untreated or treated with metoprolol (50 mg twice daily, up to 200 mg daily) and hydralazine (25 mg twice daily, up to 150 mg daily)[62]. Induction of labour because of maternal or fetal complications was more frequent in the untreated group of patients. Proteinuria occurred in five untreated and in nine treated patients. There was one perinatal death in the untreated group and three in the treated group. Birth weight was not significantly different between the two groups, nor were bradycardia, respiratory distress syndrome and hypoglycaemia. About 29% of the untreated patients had to be delivered or given antihypertensive therapy because of a severe increase in blood pressure, while only 11% of the treated patients required urgent delivery for the same reason. The authors concluded that treatment with metoprolol and hydralazine reduced the risk of severe increases in blood pressure and the consequent need for urgent delivery[62].

Acebutolol

This cardioselective β-blocking drug crosses the placenta and is known to cause neonatal hypotension[65]. In an uncontrolled study in which the effects on the neonate of acebutolol given to pregnant women

207

(200–800 mg daily; 10 cases) were compared with methyldopa (500–750 mg daily; 10 cases), acebutolol was found to cause a significant decrease in both neonatal systolic blood pressure and neonatal heart rate. This effect lasted at least 3 days (the neonates were not followed for longer periods). Blood glucose was not significantly affected[66].

Atenolol

Atenolol is used in pregnancy in a dosage of 50–100 mg per day[1]. A randomized, double-blind prospective study with atenolol has been performed in 120 pregnant women with pregnancy-induced hypertension; atenolol was compared with placebo[67]. The drug, given once daily, was effective in correcting hypertension at a daily dosage of 100 mg in 17 women and 200 mg in the remainder. Growth retardation, neonatal hypoglycaemia, respiratory distress syndrome, and hyperbilirubinaemia were observed as often in the atenolol group as in the placebo treated group. Only neonatal bradycardia was more frequent in neonates exposed to atenolol, but caused no clinical problems[67].

In conclusion, both maternal and neonatal responses to therapy with β-blockers were excellent. Unfortunately, the available prospective controlled studies have been performed in heterogeneous populations which included patients with both pregnancy-induced hypertension and essential hypertension, so that it is difficult to know whether the good results occurred in either or both of these types of hypertension[53]. Furthermore, the long-term effects on the growing child have still to be evaluated[36].

Labetalol

Labetalol is a sympathetic blocking agent that is unique in having both α- and β-blocking properties. It is now widely used for treating hypertension and has also been used in pregnancy both for oral long-term treatment (in a recent survey it was selected as the drug of first choice by 8% of the respondents)[68] and for emergency therapy intravenously.

Oral labetalol has been used for treating both PIH and CHP, in doses between 300 and 900 mg (up to 1200 mg) daily[69]. The safety of the drug with respect to maternal and perinatal outcome has been established.

After intravenous injection (1 mg per kg bodyweight), labetalol has been shown to decrease blood pressure promptly without causing maternal tachycardia, headache, or other side-effects[70–73]. Although the drug does not affect placental or fetal blood flow[74] or fetal heart rate[75], side effects have been suspected in neonates[76], since it is known to cross the placenta. This point has been examined recently by serially measuring systolic blood pressure, heart and respiratory rates, palmar sweating, blood glucose and metabolic and vasomotor responses to cold stress, over the first 72 hours of life, in 22 term infants, 11 of whom were born to mothers treated (for at least 7 days up to 20 weeks) with labetalol (100–300 mg three times daily) and 11 born to untreated mothers[77]. Infants of treated mothers showed only a mild transient hypotension that had no clinical significance and disappeared within 24 hours; it is concluded that labetalol does not cause clinically important sympathetic blockade in the mature newborn babies, so that no precautions are necessary in infants whose mothers have received the drug before delivery[77]. The safety of the drug for the newborns may be due to two factors: (a) labetalol is rapidly excreted, and (b) the combined α- and β-receptor blocking properties counteract each other[77].

Hydralazine

Hydralazine has been widely used to treat both PIH and CHP, for acute therapy both by intravenous or intramuscular administration, and orally at a dosage of 50–200 mg daily[1]. Reductions in blood pressure and systemic vascular resistance seem more prominent in patients with PIH than in those with CHP[78]. The drug causes vasodilatation by a direct effect on peripheral arterioles. Cerebral blood flow and intracranial pressure increase[79,80] thereby accounting for the frequent occurrence of headache. Reflex tachycardia in response to vasodilatation is also frequent and may exaggerate the physiological hyperdynamic state of pregnancy. Other side-effects of hydralazine, restlessness, anxiety, nausea, vomiting and epigastric pain may mimic impending eclampsia[36].

Hydralazine reduces placental function in pregnant women with chronic hypertension[81] and has been reported to cause fetal growth retardation[82,83]. Since the vasodilatation caused by hydralazine is responsible for an increase in sympathetic tone that may cause a reduction in placental blood flow, Redman[36] has suggested using hydralazine in patients already on methyldopa; this may retard the sympathetically mediated response to the drug, thereby preventing fetal distress. It is also used in association with β-blockers or with clonidine.

Calcium antagonists

The contraction of skeletal, smooth, and cardiac muscle cells depends on the increased intracellular concentration of calcium ions. Drugs that block the inward calcium ion current from the extracellular space are referred to as calcium antagonists.

Nifedipine is a drug with selective activity for vascular cells. It has, therefore, been widely used in recent years for treating hypertension. Up to now there is only one report on the use of nifedipine in pregnancy-associated hypertension[84]. When given orally (5–10 mg) to 21 women with acute episodes of severe hypertension in the peripartum period, nifedipine induced a decrease in blood pressure of 26/20 mmHg which occurred within 20 minutes and lasted at least 4 hours; the hypotensive effect was not potentiated by concurrent administration of other antihypertensive drugs (contrary to the observation in non-pregnant patients). No adverse effects were observed in the fetuses and maternal side-effects were mainly headache, palpitation and cutaneous flushing[84,85]. The drug is also used to suppress premature uterine activity[85].

Magnesium ions may potentiate the effects of calcium antagonists[86]. This is important when using calcium antagonists in patients treated with magnesium sulphate for eclampsia[36].

210

Methyldopa

Despite some studies showing fetal growth retardation[43,61] methyldopa remains the best and safest antihypertensive drug for treating hypertension in pregnant women[36,38]. In a recent survey among obstetricians, methyldopa was selected as the first-choice drug for treating hypertension by 75% of the respondents[68]. Prolonged treatment of severe hypertension with methyldopa in pregnancy has been successful. Controlled trials of methyldopa given either alone or with a diuretic for mild hypertension in pregnancy have resulted in improved perinatal outcome. Treatment of mild hypertension with methyldopa also reduces the frequency of severe hypertensive episodes during gestation. The drug is used at the dosage recommended for non-pregnant patients (from 750 mg up to 4 g daily)[36].

Methyldopa crosses the placenta and is found in fetal plasma. Neonatal blood pressure after maternal treatment is significantly reduced, but becomes normal within the first 5 days of life[87].

Long-term follow-up reports (up to $7\frac{1}{2}$ years from birth) are available on 195 children who entered a randomly controlled trial of the effect of methyldopa on growth and development. The data demonstrated no significant differences between children of treated mothers and children of untreated mothers in standing and supine blood pressures or in mean intelligence quotient despite a reduction in head circumference in sons whose mothers entered the trial between weeks 16 and 20 of gestation[88].

Clonidine

Clonidine exerts its major effect via the central nervous system. In addition, it stimulates the vagal nuclei, thereby slowing the heart rate. Thus, clonidine is useful in blocking the reflex tachycardia due to hydralazine or diazoxide. A questionnaire survey carried out in 1978 in the U.K. and Ireland showed that 21.1% of 1093 obstetricians would continue clonidine when a patient with moderately severe hypertension became pregnant. In another recent survey among obstetricians, 4% of the respondents suggested clonidine as the drug of first choice[68].

Recently, a prospective double-blind, randomized controlled trial has been carried out to compare clonidine (150–1500 μg per day in 2–4 divided doses) with methyldopa (250 mg up to 2 g daily) in 100 pregnant women with hypertension[89]. Eleven out of 47 patients treated with clonidine had essential hypertension (the others had pregnancy-induced hypertension). The results indicate that the two drugs have a similar effect on blood pressure, maternal morbidity and fetal mortality: in particular there was neither significant neonatal hypotension nor rebound hypertension in either group. It was concluded that clonidine is as effective as methyldopa in treating hypertension in pregnancy, without significant adverse effects in the neonatal period[89].

Ketanserin

Ketanserin is a serotonin antagonist that competitively and selectively blocks serotoninergic receptors, thereby being effective in treating PIH. The drug is currently under investigation. In a recent study, ketanserin was given intravenously in 10 or 20 mg boluses to 16 patients with severe preeclampsia in labour. Systolic and diastolic blood pressures were lowered significantly; maternal heart rate was unchanged, but fetal rate increased slightly[90].

Converting enzyme inhibitors

The renin–angiotensin system is stimulated during gestation. Plasma renin activity increases early in normal pregnancy; the consequent increase in aldosterone compensates for the natriuretic effect of progesterone. Although plasma renin in pregnancy is primarily of renal origin, the high concentration of renin in uterus, placenta and amniotic fluid makes these sites potential sources of additional renin in pregnancy[2]. The role of uterine renin in the physiology of pregnancy remains unknown. It is suggested that it plays an important role in regulating uterine blood flow by increasing angiotensin II and, through angiotensin II, the uterine PGE2 synthesis; PGE2 will decrease uterine vascular resistance, thereby increasing uterine blood flow[2]. The administration of captopril to pregnant rabbits reduced uterine blood flow without changing cardiac output or renal blood flow[91] while at the same time it decreased the PGE level in the uterine vein[2]. Fetal mortality in pregnant rabbits treated with captopril was almost 100%, despite there being no change in systemic blood pressure[91,92]. A fetal renin–angiotensin system is detectable after 5 weeks of pregnancy; it is greatly stimulated during delivery.

The administration of a converting enzyme inhibitor (e.g. captopril) to a pregnant woman will therefore inhibit maternal, placental and fetal renin–angiotensin systems. Since vascular senstitivity to angiotensin II is increased in preeclampsia, it was assumed that captopril would have a beneficial effect in hypertensive pregnant women, at least in PIH. On the contrary, the drug has been reported to have disastrous effects on fetal survival in several species[93,94], possibly through its effect on uterine blood flow.

Only a few cases of pregnant women treated with captopril have been reported in recent literature. One of these cases was a 47-year-old woman whose hypertension had been under control for a long time with a combination of chlorthalidone (25 mg daily), sotalol (160 mg daily), captopril (150 mg daily) and a low-salt diet. Amenorrhoea for 5 months was interpreted as menopause; when pregnancy was diagnosed, captopril was not withdrawn because of the risk of uncontrolled hypertension. Intrauterine growth retardation was observed; after 36 weeks of gestation, a small girl was delivered by caesarean section. Captopril was measured but was undetectable in umbilical cord blood[95].

Another case was that of a 22-year-old woman treated with captopril (100 mg daily) and diuretics because of nephrotic syndrome and hypertension. When she became pregnant, diuretics were stopped and acebutolol (400 mg daily) was added to captopril. Intrauterine growth retardation was also observed in this case; after 34 weeks of gestation a small boy was delivered by caesarean section. The baby needed artificial ventilation, had frequent episodes of hypotension (probably related to acebutolol, which crosses the placenta) for 10 days and had a patent ductus arteriosus that required surgical closure[65]. This abnormality has been reported in two more cases[96]; it has been attributed to captopril stimulating release of prostaglandins, PGE2 in particular[65,97].

In a recent review of worldwide literature, 15 cases of hypertensive women treated with captopril are discussed, including seven new cases[97]. The outcome of these pregnancies was one spontaneous and two therapeutic abortions, one intrauterine death after 28 weeks of gestation and two deaths with neonatal anuria. The remaining nine pregnancies were successful, with delivery or caesarian section before term in 8 cases (three cases of neonatal respiratory distress) and with birth at term of twins in one. In 13 cases the mother was treated because of renal or essential hypertension; in only two cases (pregnancies ended in intrauterine death and neonatal death with anuria) was captopril given (with propranolol, clonidine, hydralazine and with frusemide, atenolol, methyldopa, hydralazine respectively) because of preeclampsia. Captopril was used alone in only two cases (one for renal hypertension and one for essential hypertension), and in both the babies survived[97]. In the two cases resulting in death with neonatal anuria, captopril was given with frusemide. It is possible that neonatal hypotension was responsible for the anuria; but it is also possible that anuria was due to the association of captopril with a diuretic (salt depletion in a premature newborn), as has been reported in the recent adult literature[98].

On the basis of experimental studies in animals and the reported results in humans, we may conclude that converting enzyme inhibitors, captopril and enalapril, should never be used in pregnancy.

Ganglion-blocking agents

Ganglion-blocking agents should not be used in pregnancy. They may cause meconium ileus in the fetus.

ACKNOWLEDGEMENT

This work was supported, in part, by CNR (Consiglio Nazionale delle Richerche, Italy), contract 78.01958.04, and by Ministero della Pubblica Istruzione (1981, 60% and 1985, 40%).

Portions of this chapter are taken from 'Treatment of Chronic Hypertension in Pregnancy' in 'The Kidney in Pregnancy', V. E.

Andreucci (Ed.), Martinus Nijhoff, Boston, 1986, and are published with the permission of the author and publisher.

References

1. Lindheimer, M. D. and Katz, A. I. (1985). Hypertension in pregnancy. *N. Engl. J. Med.*, **313,** 675–80
2. Gregorini, G., Perico, N. and Remuzzi, G. (1986). Pathogenesis of preeclampsia. In Andreucci, V. E. (Ed.) *The Kidney in Pregnancy* pp. 13–33. (Boston: Martinus Nijhoff)
3. Gant, N. F., Pritchard, J. A. (1986). Hypertension complicating pregnancy. In Andreucci, V. E. (Ed.), *The Kidney in Pregnancy*, pp. 95–121. (Boston: Martinus Nijhoff)
4. Petrucco, O. M., Thomson, N. M., Lawrence, J. R. and Weldon, M. W. (1974). Immunofluorescent studies in renal biopsies in pre-eclampsia. *Br. Med. J.*, **1,** 473–6
5. McKillop, C., Forbes, C. D, Howie, P. W. and Prentice, C. R. M. (1976). Soluble fibrinogen/fibrin complexes in pre-eclampsia. *Lancet*, **1,** 56–48
6. Scott, J. R., Beer, A. E. and Stastny, P. (1976). Immunogenetic factors in pre-eclampsia and eclampsia. *J. Am. Med. Assoc.*, **235,** 402–4
7. Stirrat, G. M., Redman, O. W. G. and Levinsky, R. J. (1978). Circulating immune complexes in pre-eclampsia. *Br. Med. J.*, **1,** 1450–1
8. Beer, A. E. (1978). Possible immunologic bases of preeclampsia/eclampsia. *Semin. Perinatol.*, **2,** 39–59
9. Strickland, D. M., Guzick, D. S., Cox, K., Gant, N. F and Rosenfeld, C. R. (1986). The relationship between abortion in the first pregnancy and development of pregnancy-induced hypertension in the subsequent pregnancy. *Am. J. Obstet. Gynecol.*, **154,** 146–8
10. MacGillivray, I. (1958). Some observations on the incidence of preeclampsia. *J. Obstet. Gynaecol. Br. Emp.*, **65,** 536–9
11. Gleicher, N. Boler, L. R Jr., Norusis, M. and Dal Granado A. (1986). Hypertensive diseases of pregnancy and parity. *Am. J. Obstet. Gynecol.*, **154,** 1044–9
12. Bonnar, J., McNicol, G. P. and Douglas A. S. (1971). Coagulation and fibrinolytic systems in preeclampsia and eclampsia. *Br. Med. J.*, **2,** 12–6
13. Wardle, E. N. (1978). Pre-eclamptic toxemia: a reappraisal. *Nephron*, **20,** 241–7
14. Abdul-Karim, R. and Assal, N. S. (1961). Pressor response to angiotensin in pregnant and nonpregnant women. *Am. J. Obstet. Gynecol.*, **82,** 246–51
15. Everett, R. B., Worley, R. J., MacDonald, P. C. and Gant, N. F. (1978). Effect of prostaglandin synthetase inhibition on pressor response to angiotensin II in human pregnancy. *J. Clin. Endocrinol. Metab.*, **46,** 1007–10
16. Remuzzi, G., Marchesi, D., Zoja, C., Muratore, D., Mecca, G., Misiani, R., Rossi, E., Barbato, M., Capetta, P, Donati, M. B. and de Gaetano, G. (1980). Reduced umbilical and placental vascular prostacyclin in severe pre-eclampsia. *Prostaglandin*, **20,** 105–10
17. Remuzzi, G., Marchesi, D. and Mecca, G. (1980). Reduction of fetal vascular prostacyclin activity in preeclampsia. *Lancet*, **2,** 310
18. Bussolino, F., Benedetto, C., Massobrio, M. and Caumussi, G. (1980). Maternal

vascular prostacyclin activity in pre-eclampsia. *Lancet*, **2**, 702

19. Downing, I., Shepherd, G. L. and Lewis, P. J. (1980). Reduced prostacyclin production in pre-eclampsia. *Lancet*, **2**, 1374

20. Carreras, L. O., Defreyn, G., Van Houtte, E., Vermylen, J. and Van Assche, A. (1981). Prostacyclin and preeclampsia. *Lancet*, **1**, 422

21. Stuart, M. J., Clark, D. A., Sunbderji, S. G., Allen, J. B., Yambo, T., Elrad, H. and Slott, J. H. (1981). Decreased prostacyclin production: a characteristic of chronic placental insufficiency syndromes. *Lancet*, **1**, 1126–8

22. Walsh, S. W. (1985). Pre-eclampsia: an inbalance in placental prostacyclin and thromboxane pathway in normotensive and hypertensive pregnancies with insufficient fetal growth. *Am. J. Obstet. Gynecol.*, **152**, 335–40

23. Wallenburg, H. C. S. and Rotmans, N. (1982). Enhanced reactivity of the platelet thromboxane pathway in normotensive and hypertensive pregnancies with insufficient fetal growth. *Am. J. Obstet. Gynecol.*, **44**, 523–8

24. Wallenburg, H. C. S., Dekker, G. A., Makovitz, J. W. and Rotmans, P. (1986). Low-dose aspirin prevents pregnancy-induced hypertension and preeclampsia in angiotensin-sensitive primigravidae. *Lancet*, **1**, 1—3

25. Gant, N. F., Daley, G. L., Chand, S., Whalley, P. J. and MacDonald, P. C. (1973). A study of angiotensin II pressor response throughout primigravid pregnancy. *J. Clin. Invest.*, **52**, 2682–9

26. Gant, N. F., Hutchinson, H. T., Siiteri, P. K. and MacDonald, P. C. (1971). Study of the metabolic clearance rate of dehydroepiandrosterone-sulfate in pregnancy. *Am. J. Obstet. Gynecol.*, **111**, 555–62

27. Pritchard, J. A., MacDonald, P. C. and Gant, N. F. (1984, 17th Edn.). Williams *Textbook of obstetrics*. Appleton-Century-Crofts, New York.

28. Chesley, L. C., Annitto, J. E. and Congrove, R. A. (1976). Long-term follow-up study of eclamptic women: sixth periodic report. *Am. J. Obstet. Gynecol.*, **124**, 446–59

29. Tillman, A. J. B. (1955). The effect of normal and toxemic pregnancy on blood pressure. *Am. J. Obstet. Gynecol.*, **70**, 589–603

30. Svensson, A. (1985) Hypertension in pregnancy. State of the art lecture. *J. Hypertension*, **3** (Suppl. 3), S395–S403

31. Svensson, A. (1985) Hypertension in pregnancy – Long-term effects on blood pressure in mothers and children. *Acta. Med. Scand.*, Suppl. 695: 5–50

32. Svensson, A., Andersch, B. and Hansson, L. (1983). Prediction of later hypertension following a hypertensive pregnancy. *J. Hypertension*, **1** (Suppl. 2), 94–6

33. Svensson, A., Andersch, B. and Hansson, L. (1985). Hypertension in pregnancy. Analysis of 261 consecutive cases. *Acta. Med. Scand.*, (Suppl. 693), 33–9

34. Svensson, A., Sigstrom, L., Andersch, B. and Hansson, L. (1984). Low erythrocyte $Na^+/K+$ ratio in children with mild blood pressure elevation and a positive family history of hypertension. *J. Hypertension*, **2** (Suppl. 3), 473–5

35. Higgins, M., Keller, J., Moore, F., Ostrander, L., Metzner, H. and Stock, L. (1980). Studies of blood pressure in young people and its relationship to personal and familial characteristics and complication of pregnancy in mothers. *Am. J. Epidemiol.*, **111**, 142–55

36. Redman, C. W. G. (1984). The management of hypertension in pregnancy. *Semin. Nephrol.*, **4**, 270–82

37. Kraus, G. W., Marchese, J. R. and Yen, S. S. C. (1966). Prophylactic use of hydrochlorothiazide in pregnancy. *J. Am. Med,. Assoc.*, **198**, 1150–4

38. Andreucci, V. E., Dal Canton, A. and Russo, D. (1986). Treatment of chronic hypertension in pregnancy. In Andreucci, V. E. (Ed.) *The Kidney in Pregnancy*, pp. 123–31. (Boston: Martinus Nijhoff)
39. Gant, N. F., Madden, J. D., Siiteri, P. K. and MacDonald, P. C. (1975). The metabolic clearance rate of dehydroisoandrosterone sulfate. III The effect of thiazide diuretics in normal and future preeclamptic pregnancies. *Am. J. Obstet. Gynecol.*, **123**, 159—63
40. Dudley, D. K. L. (1985). Minibolus diazoxide in the management of severe hypertension in pregnancy. *Am. J. Obstet. Gynecol.*, **151**, 196–200
41. Chesley, L. C. (1978). *Hypertensive disorders in pregnancy*, New York: Appleton-Century-Crofts
42. Page, E. P and Christiansen, R. (1976). Influence of blood pressure changes with and without proteinuria upon outcome of pregnancy. *Am. J. Obstet. Gynecol.*, **126**, 821–9
43. Mabie, W. C., Pernoll, M. L. and Biswas, M. K. (1986). Chronic hypertension in pregnancy. *Obstet. Gynecol.*, **67**, 197–205
44. Sibai, B. M. and Anderson, G. D. (1986). Pregnancy outcome of intensive therapy in severe hypertension in first trimester. *Obstet. Gynecol.*, **67**, 517–22
45. Strandgaard, S., Olesen, J. and Skinhoj, E. (1973). Autoregulation of brain circulation in severe arterial hypertension. *Br. Med. J.*, **1**, 507–10
46. Strandgaard S. (1976) Autoregulation of cerebral blood flow in hypertensive patients: the modifying influence of prolonged antihypertensive treatment in the tolerance to acute, drug-induced hypotension. *Circulation*, **53**, 720–7
47. Chamberlain, G. V. P., Lewis, P. J., De Swiet, M. and Bulpitt, C. J. (1978). How obstetricians manage hypertension in pregnancy. *Br. Med. J.*, **1**, 626–9
48. Nolten, W. E. and Ehrlich, E. N. (1986). Sodium metabolism in normal pregnancy and in preeclampsia. In Andreucci, V. E. (Ed.). *The Kidney in Pregnancy*, pp. 81–94. (Boston: Martinus Nijhoff)
49. Christianson, R. and Page, E. W. (1976). Diuretic drugs and pregnancy. *Obstet. Gynecol.*, **48**, 647–52
50. Suoni, S., Saarikoski, S., Tahvanainen, K., Paakkonen, A. and Olkkonne, H. (1985). Acute effects of dihydralazine mesylate, furosemide and metoprolol on maternal hemodynamics in pregnancy-induced hypertension. *Am. J. Obstet. Gynecol.*, **155**, 122–5
51. Davison, J. M. (1986). Renal function during normal pregnancy and the effect of renal disease and preeclampsia. In Andreucci, V. E. (Ed.). *The Kidney in Pregnancy*, pp. 65–80. (Boston: Martinus Nijhoff)
52. Robinson, M. (1958). Salt in pregnancy. *Lancet*, **I**, 178–81
53. Rubin, R. C. (1981). Beta-blockers in pregnancy. *N. Engl. J. Med.*, **305**, 1323–6
54. Harden, T. P. and Stander, R. W. (1968). Effects of adrenergic blocking agents and catecholamines in human pregnancy. *Am. J. Obstet. Gynecol.*, **102**, 226–35
55. Redman, C. W. G. (1980) Treatment of hypertension in pregnancy. *Kidney Int.*, **18**, 267–78
56. Tcherdakoff, P., Colhard, M., Berrard, E., Kraft, C., Dupay, A. and Bernante, J. M. (1978). Propranolol in hypertension during pregnancy. *Br. Med. J.*, **2**, 670
57. Eliahou, H. E., Silverberg, D. S., Reisin, E., Romem, I., Mashrach, S. and Serr, D. M. (1978). Propranolol for the treatment of hypertension in pregnancy. *Br. J. Obstet. Gynecol.*, **85**, 431–6
58. Bott-Kanner, G., Schweitzer, A., Reisner, S. H., Joel-Cohen, S. J. and Rosenfeld,

J. B. (1980). Propranolol and hydralazine in the management of essential hypertension in pregnancy. *Br. J. Obstet. Gynecol.*, **87**, 110–4

59. Lieberman, B. A., Stirrat, G. M., Cohen, S. L., Beard, R. W., Pinker, G. D. and Belsey, E. (1978). The possible adverse effect of propranolol on the fetus in pregnancies complicated by severe hypertension. *Br. J. Obstet. Gynecol.*, **85**, 678–83

60. Fidler, J., Smith, V., Fayers, P. and de Swiet, M. (1983). Randomized controlled comparative study of methyldopa and oxprenolol in treatment of hypertension in pregnancy. *Br. Med. J.*, **286**, 1927–30

61. Gallery, E. D. M., Ross, M. R. and Gyory, A. Z. (1985). Antihypertensive treatment in pregnancy: analysis of different responses to oxprenolol and methyldopa. *Br. Med. J.*, **291**, 563–6

62. Hogstedt, S., Lindeberg, S., Axelsson, O., Lindmark, G., Rane, A., Sandstrom, B. and Linberg, B. S. (1985). A prospective controlled trial of metoprolol-hydralazine treatment in hypertension during pregnancy. *Acta Obstet. Gynecol. Scand.*, **64**, 505–10

63. Lim, Y. L. and Walters, W. A. W. (1979). Hemodynamics of mild hypertension in pregnancy. *Br. J. Obstet. Gynecol.*, **86**, 198–204

64. Sandstrom, B. O. (1978). Antihypertensive treatment with the adrenergic beta-receptor blocker metoprolol during pregnancy. *Gynecol. Obstet. Invest.*, **9**, 195–204

65. Boutroy, M. J., Vert, P., Hurault de Ligny, B. and Miton, A. (1984) (letter). Captopril administration in pregnancy impairs fetal angiotensin converting enzyme activity and neonatal adaptation. *Lancet*, **2**, 935–6

66. Dumez, Y., Tchobroutsky, C., Hornych, H. and Amiel-Tison, C. (1981). Neonatal effects of maternal administration of acebutolol. *Br. Med. J.*, **283**, 1077–9

67. Rubin, P. C., Clark, D. M., Summer, D. J., Low, R. A., Butters, L. and Reynolds B. (1983). Placebo controlled trial of atenolol in treatment of pregnancy-associated hypertension. *Lancet*, **1**, 431–4

68. Trudinger, B. J. and Parik, I. (1982). Attitudes to the management of hypertension in pregnancy: a survey of Australian fellows. *Aust. N.Z. J. Obstet. Gynecol.*, **22**, 191

69. Lardoux, H., Blazquez, G., Leperlier, E., Chouty, F. and Gerard, J. (1986). Le labetolol dans le traitement de l'hypertension arterielle gravidique. *Presse Med.*, **15**, 759–60

70. Lamming, G. D., Broughton Pipkin, F. and Seymond, E. M. (1980). Comparison of the alpha and beta blocking drug labetalol, and methyldopa in the treatment of moderate and severe pregnancy-induced hypertension. *Clin. Exp. Hypertension*, **2**, 865–95

71. Lunell, N. O., Hjemdahl, P., Fredholm, B. B., Nisell, H., Persson, B. and Wager, J. (1981). Circulatory and metabolic effects of a combined alpha- and beta-adrenoceptor blocker (labetalol) in hypertension of pregnancy. *Br. J. Clin. Pharmacol.*, **12**, 345–8

72. Garden, A., Davey, D. A. and Dommisse, J. (1982). Intravenous labetalol and intravenous dihydralazine in severe hypertension in pregnancy. *Clin. Exp. Hypertension*, **1**, 371–83

73. Rubin, P. C., Butters, L. and Kelman, K. W. (1983). Labetalol disposition and concentration-effect relationship during pregnancy. *Br. J. Clin. Pharmacol.*, **15**, 465–70

74. Jouppila, P., Kirkinen, P., Koivula, A. and Ylikorkala, O. (1986). Labetalol does

not alter the placental and fetal blood flow or maternal prostanoids in pre-eclampsia. *Br. J. Obstet. Gynecol.*, **93**, 543–7

75. Lunell, N. O., Nylund, L. and Lewander, R. (1982). Acute effect of an anti-hypertensive drug, labetalol, on uteroplacental blood flow. *B. J. Obstet. Gynecol.*, **89**, 640–4

76. Woods, D. L. and Malan, A. F. (1983). Side effects of labetalol in newborn infants. *Br. J. Obstet. Gynecol.*, **90**, 876

77. MacPherson, M., Broughton Pipkin, F. and Rutter, N. (1986). The effect of maternal labetalol on the newborn infant. *Br. J. Obstet. Gynecol.*, **93**, 539–42

78. Kuzniar, J., Skret, A., Piela, A., Szmigiel, Z. and Zaczek, T. (1985). Hemodynamic effects of intravenous hydralazine in pregnant women with severe hypertension. *Obstet. Gynecol.*, **66**, 453–8

79. McCall, M. L. (1953). Cerebral circulation and metabolism in toxemia of pregnancy: observations on the effects of veratrum viride and apresoline (1-hydrazinophthalazine). *Am. J. Obstet. Gynecol.*, **66**, 1015–30

80. Overgaard, J. and Skinhoj, E. (1975). A paradoxical cerebral hemodynamic effect of hydralazine. *Stroke*, **6**, 402–4

81. Gant, N. F., Madden, J. D., Siiteri, P. K. and MacDonald, P. C. (1976). The metabolic clearance rate of dehydroisoandrosterone sulfate. IV Acute effects of induced hypertension, hypotensin and natriuresis in normal and hypertensive pregnancies. *Am. J. Obstet. Gynecol.*, **124**, 143–8

82. Vink, G. J., Moodley, J. and Philport, R. H. (1980). Effect of dihydralazine on the fetus in the treatment of maternal hypertension. *Obstet. Gynecol.*, **55**, 519–22

83. Vink, G. J. and Moodley, J. (1982). The effect of low-dose dihydralazine on the fetus in the emergency treatment of hypertension in pregnancy. *S. Afr. Med. J.*, **62**, 475–7

84. Walters, B. N. J. and Redman, C. W. G. (1984). Treatment of severe pregnancy-associated hypertension with the calcium antagonist nifedipine. *Br. J. Obstet. Gynecol.*, **91**, 330–6

85. Read, M. D. and Wellby, D. E. (1986). The use of a calcium antagonist (nifedipine) to suppress preterm labor. *Br. J. Obstet. Gynecol.*, **93**, 933–7

86. Turlapaty, P. D. M., Weiner, R. and Altura, B. M. (1981). Interaction of magnesium and verapamil on tone and contractility of vascular smooth muscle. *Eur. J. Pharmacol.*, **74**, 263–72

87. Whitelaw, A. (1981). Maternal methyldopa treatment and neonatal blood pressure. *Br. Med. J.*, **283**, 471

88. Cockburn, J., Moar, V. A., Dunsted, M. and Redman C. W. G. (1982). Final report of study on hypertension during pregnancy: the effects of specific treatment on the growth and development of the children. *Lancet*, **1**, 647–9

89. Horvath, J. S., Phippard, A., Korda, A., Henderson-Smart, D. J., Child, A. and Tiller, D. J. (1985). Clonidine hydrochloride – A safe and effective anti-hypertensive agent in pregnancy. *Obstet. Gynecol.*, **66**, 634–8

90. Hulme, V. A. and Odendaal, J. (1986). Intrapartum treatment of preeclamptic hypertension by ketanserin. *Am. J. Obstet. Gynecol.*, **155**, 260–2

91. Ferris, T. F and Weir, E. K. (1983). Effect of captopril on uterine blood flow and prostaglandin E synthesis in the pregnant rabbit. *J. Clin. Invest.*, **71**, 809–15

92. Broughton Pipkin, F., Turner, S. R. and Symond E. M. (1980). Possible risk with captopril in pregnancy: some animal data. *Lancet*, **1**, 1256

93. Broughton Pipkin, F., Symonds, E. M. and Turner, S. R. (1982). The effect of

219

captopril (SQ 14.225) upon mother and fetus in the chronically cannulated ewe and in the pregnant rabbit. *J. Physiol.*, **323**, 415–22

94. Keith, I. M., Will, J. A. and Weir, E. K. (1982). Captopril association with fetal death and pulmonary vascular changes in the rabbit. *Proc. Soc. Exp. Biol. Med.*, **170**, 378–83

95. Fiocchi, R., Lijnen, P., Fagard, R., Staessen, J., Amery, A., Van Assche, F., Spitz, B. and Rademaker, M. (1984) (letter). Captopril during pregnancy. *Lancet*, **2**, 1153

96. Caraman, P. ., Miton, A., Hurualt de Ligny, B., Kessler, M., Boutroy, M., Schwetzer, M., Brocard, O., Ragage, J. P. and Netter, P. (1984). Grossesses sous captopril. *Therapie*, **39**, 59–62

97. Plouin, P. F. and Tchobroutsky, C. (1985). Inhibition de l'enzyme de conversion de l'angiotensine au cours de la grossesse humaine. *Presse Med.*, **14**, 2175–8

98. Andreucci, V. E., Conte, G., Dal Canton, A., Di Minno, G. and Usberti, M. (1987). The causal role of salt depletion in acute renal failure due to captopril in hypertensive patients with a single functioning kidney and renal artery stenosis. *Renal Failure*, **10**, 9–20

INDEX